How Stress and Anxiety Impact Your Decision Making

MAKING BETTER DECISIONS.
DRIVING BETTER OUTCOMES.

Steven Howard

Caliente Press

How Stress and Anxiety Impact Your Decision Making
Making Better Decisions.
Driving Better Outcomes.

Copyright ©2020 by Steven Howard

ISBN: 978-1-943702-15-2 (print edition)
    978-1-943702-16-9 (Kindle edition)

All rights reserved. No part of this publication may be reproduced, distributed or transmitted in any form or by any means, including photocopying, recording, or other electronic or mechanical methods, without the prior written permission of the publisher, except in the case of brief quotations embodied in critical reviews and certain other noncommercial uses permitted by copyright law. For permission requests, write to the publisher, addressed "Attention: Permissions Coordinator," at the address below.

Published by:
Caliente Press
1775 E Palm Canyon Drive, Suite 110-198
Palm Springs, CA 92264
www.CalientePress.com
Email: steven@CalientePress.com

Cover Design: Héctor Castañeda

ENDORSEMENTS AND PRAISE

Steven's latest book is timely as the world transitions to a post-pandemic space teeming with mounting anxiety and stress for many. It is amazing how Steven packed so many useful tips and techniques along with supporting scientific facts and interesting anecdotes into this practical and easy-to-read guidebook.

Joe Locetta
Leadership and Life Coach and Author

The choices we make directly affect our moment-to-moment experiences. When we become aware and take responsibility for our choices we also become the guide of our own well-being.

Steven's book *How Stress and Anxiety Impact Your Decision Making* is a wonderful resource for mindful techniques that will guide you into living well. A life is based on self-awareness, understanding (common sense) and healthy practices.

Valeria Teles
Founder of Fit for Joy
Well-Being Author, Coach, and Podcaster

What makes a book valuable to me is when it's compelling to read, backed by research, and highly practical to implement. Steven Howard is simply brilliant and scores full marks on all these.

Thank you Steven and for another valuable contribution to the world.

Sumit Seth
Managing Director
Forum India

Steven's latest book is an insightful deep dive into the neurobiology of how and why stress and anxiety impact our cognitive decision making. By reading this book you will learn how to harness mindful decision making through greater awareness and practical strategies.

As both a leadership and mindfulness expert, with decades of coaching for global business executives and managers, Steven crystallizes the pathways to making better decisions and driving better outcomes. His writing and coaching on mindfulness thinking and mindful leadership sets a much-needed gold standard as the world recovers from the coronavirus pandemic and its aftermath.

This book shows why *how* you think is equally or more important than *what* you think.

Jennifer Bishop
Founder and Chief Mindfulness Officer
Mindful Life Training
Australia

Steven has written a book that will not only cause you to think about the way you make decisions, but also gives you a call to action. His research on how the mind reacts under stress and anxiety is insightful and forms a solid basis for how we approach key decision making in our lives.

It is a must read to improve the environment under which you make important decisions, that will then lead to better decisions and a more productive life.

Mark Harner
Author
Living Uncommonly

We are in a world that requires constant decisions and won't wait for us to feel ready. It's as simple as this: Steven clears up the path for awakening. He invites mindfulness into our lives to slow down and practice our own way towards a happier journey.

It's fantastic and really effective. Thank you, Steven!

Ayda Velasco
Specialist in human transformational process
Spiritual Coach
Columbia

This practical and insightful book is an excellent guide for everyone (not just leaders) on how to manage stress and anxiety.

Steven Howard demonstrates his deep understanding of the science and practice of mindfulness and offers practical applications for meeting today's challenges.

It is an extraordinary resource for anyone aiming to improve their overall health and achieve better decision making.

Alison Hutchens
Mindfulness Meditation Coach
Mind Body Energy
Australia

Contents

Introduction 7
Decision-Making Factors 13
Decision-Making Limitations 21
Stress Leads to Poor Thinking and Bad Decisions 39
Reducing Stress for Better Decisions and Better Outcomes 65
Mindfulness 87
The Impact of Mindfulness on Decision Making 105
Benefits of Mindfulness and Meditation 109
Shifting Into Mindfulness 123
More Mindfulness Techniques 139
Mindfulness Meditation Techniques 155
It's Up To You 165
Recommended Resources 169
About the Author 171

Dedication

Adriana Fuentes Diaz

You came into my life unexpectedly.
Touched my heart.
And changed my life forever.

The mind is like water.

*When it is turbulent, blocked or agitated
it is difficult to see clearly.*

*When it is calmed, freed and unencumbered,
everything becomes clearer.*

People are the same.

Introduction

Adults make tens of thousands of decisions a day – up to 70,000 according to some research. Many of these decisions are unconscious ones, like where to place your car keys when returning home or how hot you set the shower temperature.

Too many decisions, however, in both the workplace and in our personal lives, are made under emotional duress. When this happens, the rational control center of our brain is no longer in charge, having been replaced by the emotional control center.

What causes this to happen? Mostly stress and anxiety, though other emotions such as anger, giddiness, frustration, pride, disappointment, and elation can also cause what Daniel Goleman labeled *emotional hijacking*.

This is true in both our personal and professional lives. I am sure you have experienced situations where you said to yourself, "I was so angry I couldn't think straight." That's an example of an emotional hijacking in play.

From a workplace perspective, stress, anxiety, pressure, deadlines, tiredness, and our relationships with co-workers can all lead to various levels of emotional hijacking. Another major cause, here in the first half of 2020, is the pandemic-influenced shelter-in-place and lockdown rules creating a significant amount of prolonged stress for a considerable portion of the world's population. Neuroscientists are fully aware of the adverse effects of prolonged stress on the brain's self-regulation control center.

Unfortunately, more of us are going to learn about this as we hear about, or personally experience, the sizeable increases in alcohol abuse, binge eating, and domestic abuse that are a worrisome side effect of these pandemic policies.

Hence the purpose of this book, excerpted from my award-winning book *Better Decisions Better Thinking Better Outcomes – How to go from Mind Full to Mindful Leadership*. The main intention here is to provide a range of tips and techniques for everyone (not just leaders as was the focus of the previous book) on how to manage stress and anxiety and prevent these from impacting your decision-making processes. I also want to encourage you to become a First Responder, rather than a First Reactor, to situations, events, and people.

Here is what I mean by that. Decades ago, I learned to scuba dive and was certified as a Rescue Diver. The first thing we are taught in the Rescue Diver certification program is to "respond, not react." There is no point in reacting and immediately jumping into the water when we hear a cry for help. Rather, we get trained to first assess the situation to see what dangers might be lurking (sharks, strong currents, floating fishing nets, etc.). Then, once we know we won't be putting ourselves, or others, in danger – and once we have ensured we have all of the appropriate gear with us – do we jump into the water and head toward the struggling person.

All this takes only a handful of seconds, but it prevents additional problems from cropping up. EMTs and others are trained to do the same, which is why they are called First Responders.

This is what we all need to do in today's world. Pause, assess the situation, and then respond, rather than react. There is too much pressure, particularly in the workplace, for fast decisions.

Leaders at all levels of organizations are compelled to make snap decisions in First Reactor mode, rather than better, more optimal decisions in First Responder mode.

So the first step to better decision making — and better outcomes — is to make the conscious and purposeful decision not to get emotionally hijacked by your overloaded brain, in order to move into a rational thinking mode.

Hence — and this is a core concept behind this book — it is not just *what* you think, but *how* you think that makes a difference in the outcomes you generate.

Another troubling long-term brain health trend is mostly produced by Generation X (those born in the years 1965 through 1979) and Millennials (those born in the years 1980 through 2000). To a much greater degree than their predecessor generations, these generations habitually engage in multitasking, live lives tethered to mobile devices, and are constantly susceptible to electronic notifications. All of those beeps, buzzes, and electronic chimes are activating unconscious stress signals in their bodies. This long-term accumulation of such constant stress is wearing down their brains, with long-term consequences for brain health and future hypertension readings.

No wonder Generation X has been identified by the American Psychological Association as the "most stressed generation in the United States."

In addition, their multitasking habits are creating brains that are losing the ability to concentrate and focus. Unfortunately, losing such capabilities is a precursor to Alzheimer's disease and other forms of dementia. The research results are clear: multitasking diminishes productivity, elevates brain fatigue, and increases stress. Yet this has become the primary operational mode for many.

These are alarming trends — for companies, organizations, and societies.

Fortunately, they are also reversible trends. But only if the leaders in companies, organizations, governments, and societies take the proper steps — first with themselves and then with their peers, employees, spouses, children, neighbors, and communities.

A few years ago, when I began to illustrate how reducing stress and increasing brain health would lead to better decisions, improved thinking and analytical capabilities, and more desirable outcomes, I immediately got the attention of the corporate and entrepreneurial worlds.

And that is what I hope to do with you, dear reader. Grab your full attention. Show you the facts about how exercise and diet impact your brain. Share with you some of the latest neuroscientific research on how mindfulness and meditation practices actually help you grow new brain neurons and increase cellular connectivity across your brain.

Perhaps most important, I also want to help you find ways to prevent emotions from hijacking your rational, cognitive resources, thus enabling you to make better decisions, think more rationally, and reduce emotional meltdowns and outbursts.

So I hope this book stirs new habits in helping you to respond cognitively, instead of emotionally react, to situations, events, and other people. I hope it arouses a desire to not only find greater peace and solitude in your life, but also to spread these messages and benefits to others.

And I hope it generates an eagerness in you to bring the concepts and ideas of this book formally into your own organization, business unit, or work team, either through the workshops my associates and I deliver or through your own enthusiastic practices and behaviors.

Together we can make your organizations less stressful, more engaging, more productive, and happier places to work. Now, wouldn't that be a wonderful outcome for you and your fellow colleagues and team members?

In the meantime, please enjoy this book and reflect on the many lessons it has to offer. The techniques described will help you make better decisions and improve your thinking prowess. They will also result in you becoming a less stressed and far healthier person.

And that, I am sure you would agree, are certainly four better outcomes that will definitely benefit you immediately, and for years to come.

Best wishes for continued success.

Steven Howard
June 2020

CHAPTER 1

Decision-Making Factors

Decisions shape our lives.

In the workplace, the decisions we make and execute also shape the lives of our team members, colleagues, direct reports, customers, suppliers, and even the communities in which we operate and live.

As humans, the decisions we make impact and shape the lives of our families, friends, neighbors, and communities.

Fortunately, decision making is a skill. And like all skills, it is something that can be learned, practiced, and enhanced over time.

Later in this book, I will share with you how mindfulness can help everyone overcome and manage their decision-making related fears and mistakes.

First, however, I want to share with you some critical factors that can impact and influence your decision making.

Your Decision-Making Brain

Scientists are gaining a grasp on the regions of the brain most responsible for our decision-making processes.

A study published in *Cell* revealed that the time it takes for the brain to create an answer to a problem correlates with the perceived difficulty of the decision and the decision-making level of cautiousness. This study, conducted by researchers at the University of Oxford, was focused on the decision threshold, which is the brain's ability to determine the level of a task based on the perceived difficulty of the task. Interestingly, our brains infer the difficulty of a task based on the initial information available to it. From this inference, the brain assigns a specified level or degree of difficulty threshold.

Intuitively, this makes sense. One of the first tasks in any decision-making process is to determine the perceived difficulty of making a viable decision. What to order at lunch at a favorite restaurant? A pretty easy decision most of the time. What to order from a restaurant in Lisbon when the menu is printed in Portuguese? That's a higher level of difficulty, unless you are fluent in Portuguese.

This study revealed one fascinating aspect of the brain's decision-making process. Apparently, the brain makes an assessment of the difficulty of a task in one single event, based on the information it initially receives. Hence, new information obtained does not, according to this study, change the perceived difficulty threshold of the decision.

Thus, based on the information absorbed at the beginning of a task or a problem to be solved, the brain determines and sets out a decision difficulty threshold in that first instant. This directly impacts how quickly or slowly a decision will be made.

It also means, in today's world of information overload, that insufficient information getting through to the brain at the start of the decision-making process is what turns relatively straightforward decisions into more difficult ones.

A lack of quality information getting through to the brain raises the perceived difficulty threshold and reduces the ability to make quicker decisions, even when timeliness is a critically important need.

The Oxford research did not look into how stress impacts the initial information received by the brain. However, other research strongly shows that stress directly impacts the prefrontal cortex, and thus is likely to impact the amount and quality of information reaching the decision-making regions of the brain.

We all know that emotions can hijack the brain's thinking processes. I believe it was psychologist and author Daniel Goleman who first described this as an "emotional hijacking." Scientists are now proving how this happens and validating mindfulness as an approach for preventing and managing emotional hijacking.

The brain comprises numerous, highly specialized modules, which are used for analyzing situations and preparing reactions to them. It is the interplay between these modules of the brain that determine behavior. Unfortunately, most of this interplay occurs subconsciously and automatically.

In a process that neuroscientists call pattern recognition, our brains reflexively try to counter decision-making anxieties by narrowing and simplifying our options. This attempt to find certainty in uncertain situations leads to premature conclusions based on previous approaches, preventing more and better options to surface or be considered.

In a similar way, emotional tagging in our memories sends us signals as to whether or not to pay attention to something or someone and what sort of action we should be considering. Interestingly, neurological research shows that when the parts of our brain controlling emotions are damaged, we become slow and incompetent decision-makers, even though we retain the capacity for objective analysis. We all know how it feels to make poor decisions when we are "emotionally hijacked."

Because some modules of the brain focus on gathering benefits and other modules concentrate on delivering benefits, your brain is often in conflict. Hence the issues people who are trying to lose weight face when they stumble upon the smell of freshly baked donuts. One part of the brain wants to gather the benefits derived from eating the donuts while another module is sending signals to reduce calorie consumption.

While these modules are interconnected, they are not integrated. Hence there are many so-called captains in the brain trying to assert command authority. While some people refer to the brain as being similar to a computer operating system, this really is not true. It is more like a collection of smartphone apps all opened at once and clamoring to be used. Just as a phone can only operate one app at a time (with the rest running in background mode), the brain only operates one module at a time with all the rest eagerly awaiting in standby mode.

These modules can also create conflict in emotional behavior. For instance, while giving someone a tongue-lashing over poor customer service may deliver an emotional benefit of expressing outrage, another brain module will be signaling that an angry outburst can have adverse effects on blood pressure and heart health. This is why people rarely feel satisfied and good after losing their temper.

The interplay of working memory and short-term memory also impacts the decision-making processes of the brain.

Working memory is task-oriented. This is how the brain creates interfaces and connections between the various processors of perception, attention, and memory. Working memory holds the information and associations relevant to a current task.

Short-term memory, on the other hand, is a cognitive process that allows us to store information (data, facts, words, sentences, concepts, etc.) for a short period of time. Short-term memory is associated with chunking, a concept that says most of us can remember about seven "chunks" of information for a brief amount of time.

When a task or decision requires a high cognitive load — the amount of mental processing power required to learn or process information — this puts a high burden on working memory. Tasks and decisions that tax our working memory capacity thus become harder to handle. Additionally, too much information, or incongruent and conflicting information, overloads short-term memory.

In either case, the decision-making brain starts to cough and sputter as cognitive stress takes over. Indecision and procrastination urges arise. Sometimes the overloaded brain triggers an emotional outburst or meltdown. In other circumstances, the brain defaults to relying on previous decisions and experiences, creating the "gut feelings" of how to proceed safely and securely, though not necessarily creatively or innovatively.

It does not take a scientific research study to acknowledge that cognitive stress interferes with creativity and innovation. We have all experienced episodes of mental fatigue caused by hits to our working memory and/or short-term memory capacities.

Fortunately, there is a readily available prescription for handling these episodes — pause, breathe, step back, take a short break, recalibrate, and then return to the task or decision-making process. Whether you need two minutes, twenty minutes, or even two hours for this mental medicine to work does not matter. You will make better decisions, and drive better outcomes, by pausing than by pushing on with a tired or overloaded brain.

Unfortunately, too many leaders and decision makers consider using this prescription to be a sign of weakness. They fear the hardness of their leadership shell will appear softened if they are seen needing to pause and take a mental refresh break. So instead, they chug on, often at a greater clip to mask their need for a recalibration pause, and rush headlong into making decisions under cognitive stress. Both their organizations and their own leadership personas suffer as a consequence.

Think of your brain in such situations as an overheated engine. Like the engine, your brain needs to cool down to function at optimal levels. Take the time you need if you want to make better decisions. Otherwise, your tired and overworked decision-making brain has no capability to produce anything except less-than-stellar decisions.

After all, numerous research studies have shown that we each have a limited amount of mental energy available to utilize when making decisions and choices. Thus, it is critical that important decisions — especially those that impact others — are made when mental energy levels are at full power.

This also explains why people tend to make poorer decisions later in the day than in the morning hours. It is a concept known as decision fatigue, and it is a common type of cognitive stress familiar to us all. There is a biological price to be paid for making decision after decision after decision all day long. The more choices made throughout the day, the harder each one becomes for an unrested and spent brain.

Similar to physical fatigue, the main difference is that most people are unaware of when they start to become low on mental energy. The problem gets escalated when an energy-depleted brain looks for shortcuts to its decision-making processing. One typical shortcut is to encourage impulsive actions that have not been thought through clearly (sure, go ahead and send that email, what could possibly go wrong?).

Another shortcut is to take the easy way out and do nothing. This saves the brain from further energy depletion as the need to agonize over options is put aside, either for a later time or forever. Doing nothing eases the mental strain of cognitive stress, but a decision to not make a decision is still a decision. And it is one with consequences and outcomes.

Sufficient and quality sleep also influence the brain's memory and decision-making functions. A recent study from researchers at the University of Zurich states that depriving ourselves of adequate sleep may lead to riskier decisions (casino operators have known this for years). Even worse, these researchers concluded that sleep shortcomings might even prevent us from realizing the increased risks from our decisions.

In the next chapter, we will explore some decision-making limitations that you are likely to encounter from time to time.

CHAPTER 2

Decision-Making Limitations

Multitasking, information overload, and constant interruptions (from both people and electronic device notifications) are negatively impairing the ways our brains work. These factors adversely impact optimal decision making. I will highlight a few of them in this chapter.

First, and perhaps the most prevalent factor, is brain fatigue and tiredness. When physical tiredness arises, we are smart enough to take a break and rest to prevent exhaustion. But what happens when mental fatigue surfaces? We push on as if being mentally tired is some sort of weakness to overcome. As a result, mental exhaustion occurs.

Mental exhaustion is a major cause of poor decision making and poor thinking. The mindfulness techniques in the chapters 8 and 9 will help you prevent mental fatigue and overcome mental exhaustion, thus putting you in a position to make better decisions and create better outcomes for you and your team.

Another major decision-making limitation is fear. In fact, weakness in decision making usually comes from a place of fear. The most common mistakes in decision making are typically caused by one of these four fears:

Fear of Taking Action — uncertainty or doubt about eventual outcomes cause many to put off making decisions. Often this is done under the disguise of wanting more information and data, a common disease known as paralysis by analysis.

Fear of Making a Mistake — many people who worry about making a decision operate from a place of insecurity. They worry about making a wrongful decision, particularly on something that should be an easy decision to make. Such insecurity builds upon itself over time, resulting in a more fearful decision-making process.

Fear of History — all of us have made mistakes and errors of judgment at some point in our lives. Unfortunately for some, the fear of repeating past mistakes weighs heavily on how some make future decisions.

Fear of Judgment —overly concerned with how others will judge them. Such people also fear how they will judge themselves, fully aware that their own self-criticisms and self-evaluations impact their personal levels of self-confidence, courage, resilience, and fortitude.

Those who are too focused on the past or the future are most prone to these decision-making fears. Being mindful, however, and bringing a focus on the present, can help prevent these four fears from surfacing and adversely impacting the decision-making process. It is also essential to understand that not making a decision is, in effect, a decision itself.

Another aspect of the decision-making process often overlooked by many concerns opportunity costs. While deliberating over options, or being delayed by fears and personal decision-making weaknesses, time is lost. This does not mean that decisions should be rushed. Far from it. However, it does mean that everyone needs to be aware of the personal fears and hurdles they bring to their decision-making process.

There is also the concept of bounded rationality. Bounded rationality is the idea that in decision making, the rationality of individuals is limited by the information they have, the cognitive limitations of their minds, and the finite amount of time they have to make a decision. Created as a theory of economic decision making by Herbert Simon, bounded rationality really defines the various limitations encountered in all decision-making efforts.

Max Bazerman and Dolly Chugh described another limitation on decision making as bounded awareness. This refers to the well-documented observation that people routinely overlook important information during the decision-making process. This is partially due to the tendency to be overly focused on the problem or task at hand, combined with our natural inclination to give greater weight to previous experiences and trusted information sources when evaluating options.

The Perils of Multitasking

Multitasking also limits our decision-making capabilities, as well as reduces our productivity levels.

A study at Stanford University revealed that regular multitasking makes it difficult for people to focus on a single task. An important finding from this study is that multitasking results in "goal-irrelevant information to compete with goal-relevant information" in the brain. The study results were quite clear: daily multitasking makes a person:

- Less effective when multitasking.

- Less effective when not multitasking.

- Less effective at prioritizing to achieve goals.

When a person multitasks, they literally reduce their intelligence levels, as measured by the ability to comprehend and understand what they are hearing and seeing. A landmark study from York University in the U.K. showed that multitaskers scored 11% lower on a standard comprehension test than those not multitasking.

The evidence is indisputable. Multitasking diminishes mental productivity, elevates brain fatigue, and increases stress. Sandra Bond Chapman, founder and chief director at the Center for BrainHealth at the University of Texas at Dallas and author of *Make Your Brain Smarter*, states frankly that multitasking is "as toxic to the brain as smoking is to the lungs."

The constant electronic notifications from computers, smartphones, and tablet devices are constantly jolting our stress hormones into action. According to endocrinologist and author Robert Lustig, these constant notifications are essentially training our brains to be in a nearly continuous state of stress and fear. In such a state, the prefrontal cortex, the part of the brain that deals with the highest-order cognitive functions, is hijacked and basically stops operating.

This results in poor decision making and regretful actions being taken since the prefrontal cortex is no longer in charge. In some ways, this state is similar to the teenage years, before the prefrontal cortex has been fully developed. Not many adults want their lives and decisions to be derived from teenage-like brains!

The keys to preventing this state of multitasking-induced stress and fear are:

1) turning off all but the most necessary notification messages, and

2) stop attempting to multitask.

Scientists have known for years what most of us refuse to admit — we really cannot multitask effectively. At least 97.5% of the population cannot, according to research. The other 2.5% have been labeled by scientists as "supertaskers," for they actually can successfully handle more than one task at a time.

So, unless you are definitely one of these elite supertaskers, most likely you can truly focus on only one thing at a time. Hence, every time you pause to check a notification message, or stop thinking about a problem or situation to answer a colleague's question, you pay a price for engaging in that interruption. It is called a "switch cost" and it automatically produces a dose of the stress hormone cortisol.

This, in turn, slows down the functioning of the prefrontal cortex and simultaneously triggers dopamine, the brain's addiction chemical. That, of course, initiates a cruel cycle of unknowingly wanting more interruptions, causing more stress and more cortisol, and then more dopamine. Hence, the desire to continue multitasking so that the longing for more dopamine can be fulfilled.

The brain can only process so much information at a time, around 50-60 bits per second, according to scientific research. The more one tries to multitask — which is really nothing more than shifting focus from one item to another since the brain can do only one thing at a time — the more this limited information processing power gets distributed across a multitude of tasks, thoughts, or data.

Battling Distractions

Another major decision-making limitation, and one which does not get adequate discussion, is the impact of unconscious bias in the decision-making process.

Decision making is fraught with biases that cloud judgment. We often remember bad experiences as good and vice versa. We can (and do) let our emotions turn a rational choice into an irrational one. And we use social cues, often unconsciously, to make choices and decisions.

According to Dr. Joseph Dispenza, author of *Evolve Your Brain*, our brains sense 400 billion bits of information per second, but we are only aware of 2,000 of those. And, according to multiple sources on the Internet, the average number of remotely conscious decisions an adult makes each day is roughly 35,000. No wonder our brain looks for shortcuts for processing all this information and making decisions.

What is bias? Bias is an assumption about a category of people, objects, and events that produces a prejudice in favor of or against a thing, person, or group. Biases may have positive or negative consequences and stem from our tendency to organize our social worlds through categorization.

While a conscious bias is explicit, an unconscious bias is implicit. Both can impact decision making, either consciously or subconsciously.

Unconscious biases are stereotypes about certain groups of people that individuals form from outside their conscious awareness. Everyone holds unconscious beliefs about various social and identity groups. In fact, unconscious biases emerge during middle childhood and appear to develop across childhood. One example of early biases most of us experienced is that girls who take charge on the school playground are labeled as "pushy" or "bossy," while boys who do the same receive praise for showing leadership capabilities.

Unconscious bias is more prevalent than conscious prejudice and is often incompatible with one's own conscious values. Additionally, unconscious bias is more likely to be predominant when we are multitasking, working under time pressure, or tired.

This universal tendency toward unconscious bias exists because bias is rooted in the brain. Scientists have recently determined that bias is located in the same region of the brain (the amygdala) associated with fear and threat.

Biases are neither good nor bad. In fact, biases allow us to efficiently process information about people. In some ways, biases are merely mental shortcuts based partially on social norms and stereotypes. Having biases does not make you (or anyone else) a bad person, but it can make you a bad decision maker.

For instance, making a decision based on a conscious or unconscious bias goes astray when we make a wrong assumption about a person and then take action or make decisions based on this wrong assumption. To avoid doing this, you need to become more aware of how your biases are influencing the decisions you make.

As Mahzarin Banaji wrote in the *Harvard Business Review*, "Most of us believe that we are ethical and unbiased. We imagine we're good decision makers, able to objectively size up a job candidate or a venture deal and reach a fair and rational conclusion that is in our, and our organization's, best interests. But more than two decades of research confirms that, in reality, most of us fall woefully short of our inflated self-perception."

Cognitive biases, which include both conscious and unconscious biases, impact the way we each see the world around us. This is neither good nor bad. It is merely an aspect of being human. The important thing is that by becoming acutely aware of our individual biases, and by understanding how our specific biases impact our own decision making, we can overcome them, or at least limit their impact if we choose to do so.

On the other hand, cognitive biases can make our judgments irrational and less objective. For instance, there is the cognitive bias known as hyperbolic discounting, which is to give more weight to the option closer to the present time when considering a trade-off between two future moments.

There is also the famous gambler's fallacy that makes a person convinced that, if a coin has landed heads up four times in a row, it is more likely to land tails up on the fifth toss. This is incorrect. On the fifth toss, the odds are still 50-50 for both heads and tails.

Unconscious biases directly influence our emotional feelings, which in turn directly impacts and sways our decision-making processes. We may think we are making rational decisions, but often we are merely rationalizing decisions based partially or majorly on emotions. As psychotherapist Kathleen Saxton says, "We may think we lead with thinking, but fundamentally what we are feeling is a greater driver."

Biases are not limited to ethnicity or gender. How prevalent are biases? They go a lot wider than you might think, as this list from the website YourBias.is shows. Each of these 24 biases can impact anyone's decision-making process:

> Self-serving bias — you believe your failures are due to external factors, yet you are responsible for your successes.
>
> Anchoring — the first thing you judge influences your judgment of all that follows.

Optimism bias — you overestimate the likelihood of positive outcomes.

Pessimism bias — you overestimate the likelihood of negative outcomes.

Negativity bias — you allow negative things to disproportionately influence your thinking.

Sunk cost — you irrationally cling to things that have already cost you something.

Group Think — you let the social dynamics of a group situation override the best outcomes.

In-group bias — you unfairly favor those who belong to your group (however you define your group).

Placebo effect — if you believe you are taking medicine, it can sometimes "work," even if it is fake.

Backfire effect—when some aspect of your core beliefs is changed, it can cause you to believe even more strongly.

Availability heuristic — your judgments are influenced by what springs to mind most readily.

Framing effect — you allow yourself to be unduly influenced by context and delivery.

Declinism — you remember the past as better than it was and expect the future to be worse than it will likely be.

Curse of knowledge — once you understand something, you presume it to be evident to everyone.

Fundamental attribution error — you judge others on their character, but yourself on the situation.

Halo effect — how much you like someone, or how attractive they are, influences your other judgments of them.

Confirmation bias — you favor things that confirm your existing beliefs.

Dunning-Kruger Effect — the more you know, the less confident you are likely to be.

Barnum Effect — you see personal specifics in vague statements by filling in the gaps.

Belief bias — if a conclusion supports your existing beliefs, you will rationalize anything that supports it.

Just-world hypothesis — your preference for justice makes you presume it exists.

Bystander effect — you presume someone else is going to do something in an emergency situation.

Reactance — you would rather do the opposite of what someone is trying to make you do.

Spotlight effect — you overestimate how much people notice how you look and act.

Memory Overload

Working memory is the short-term memory system that helps us remember things while we do a task, such as typing the URL address of a website or remembering our User ID and password access codes.

The working memory function within the brain has limited capacity, which means it can retain only a finite amount of information at any given time. Thus, if the working memory of the brain is absorbed with handling stress-related thoughts, there is less working memory capacity available to attend to the other tasks at hand, including making decisions.

If threat-stimuli information enters the brain's working memory capacity, it can exert a negative influence on subsequent thoughts, emotions, and behaviors. Again, this happens automatically and subconsciously. The antidote is to become acutely aware when this happens, and then take proactive steps such as purposeful breathing, reframing your perspectives, and preventing negative self-talk from taking over (all techniques discussed in chapters 8 and 9).

In 2008, a study from the University of California San Diego (called *How Much Information?*) reported that the average American consumed over 34 gigabytes and 100,000 words of information on a typical day. Two things should jump out at you from this data:

1) readers are not the average person and thus are likely to be exposed to a much higher amount of information, and

2) in the 12 years since this study was conducted, it is highly unlikely that the amount of information all of us is exposed to daily has decreased. So the corresponding figures for today are undoubtedly much higher.

All this information absorption and processing is taxing our finite short-term memory resources. This clutters our ability to work on tasks and make decisions. Cramming too much information into short-term memory clogs the brain. It is like having too many tabs open on a web browser, which slows down the processing speed of your computer.

But the solution does not come from trying to process this incoming information overload faster. The solution is to reduce the amount of unnecessary information stored in short-term memory.

Trying to use short-term memory for long-term memory storage can lead to chronic stress, fatigue, and numerous memory recall issues. The challenge is to stop forcing your short-term memory to store data, details, and information you won't need until later. This would free up more short-term memory and information processing power to use for making higher quality decisions.

Memory overload often triggers a feeling of brain fog, a sensation of mental confusion combined with uncertainty, temporary memory recall issues, and a befuddled wondering of why this is happening. It feels like a cloud has wrapped itself around your head, blocking your ability to think clearly and to process information as quickly as you usually do.

The critical thing to remember is that brain fog is not the problem, unless it is experienced frequently over long periods (if so, contact your doctor). Instead, brain fog is usually a symptom of other underlying problems your body and brain are struggling with: insufficient sleep, enhanced stress, multitasking, minor dehydration, improper nutritional intake, and even allergies. The cure: in addition to a momentary pause to collect yourself (purposeful breathing and a short walk outside are top tactics), the best course of action is to correct these underlying root causes through better sleep, better stress management, drinking more water, eating healthier, and focusing entirely on one task at a time.

Why Mind Full People Make Bad Decisions

The daily juggling of data, reports, email, meetings, decisions, and way too much information makes it difficult to cope and results in many of us running on autopilot. I regularly see zoned out and inattentive people struggling to cope with their never-ending to-do lists.

Many are so consumed with firefighting activities that few realize these fires were caused by the poor decisions and choices they have made. Thus the cycle of stress-induced poor decision making is perpetuated by the stress of making course corrections due to the unanticipated and undesirable results from previous poor decisions.

No wonder so many people operate in a *mind full* mode. This is not good. A more effective method is to make decisions in a mindful mode. Fortunately, this is a skill that can be learned, practiced, and ingrained.

In the workplace, leaders, managers, and supervisors get paid to make decisions and to ensure the execution of their decisions. And to course correct whenever a wrong decision is made, or unexpected results occur from what was deemed a correct decision at the time.

Outside the workplace, many folks spend an excessive amount of time in the decision-making process, deliberating the pros and cons of multiple options, analyzing potential outcomes, and trying to anticipate or measure the probable costs and impact of their decisions.

In an interview published by *Inc. Magazine* (May 2018), Stanford decision analysis expert Michelle Florendo shared five mistakes people make when facing hard choices:

1. Spending too much time in the research phase.
2. Not giving yourself enough time to learn how to make great decisions.
3. Confusing the quality of the decision with the quality of the outcome.
4. Mistaking your options as fixed and binary.
5. Getting stuck in a perfectionism trap.

Despite good intentions, everyone makes mistakes. And, unfortunately, no matter how good the information, data, and analysis available, intelligent people sometimes make important decisions that are flawed, imperfect, and even occasionally unsound.

According to neuroscientists, we make decisions mainly through two hardwired and unconscious processes called pattern recognition and emotional tagging. While these processes often formulate quick and effective decisions (particularly for routine and oft-repeated choices and determinations), there can be fallout when these methods get used for highly important decisions, especially when under stress or time pressures.

Unfortunately, pattern recognition and emotional tagging can warp the decision-making process through self-interest, emotional attachment, unconscious biases, or misleading memories. The result: errors of judgment leading to flawed, specious, and mistaken decisions that often produce unintended consequences and generally fail to produce expected outcomes.

Here's how the process works. First, the brain uses pattern recognition to assess a situation or the information available concerning a situation or problem that needs resolving. Then, based on the emotional associations (or tags) attached to any recognizable patterns, the brain helps us determine how to react (or ignore) what it has assessed.

This process of pattern recognition uses up to 30 different parts and regions of the brain to integrate and handle information. When faced with a new situation — either an event or a new problem to solve — pattern recognition helps us make assumptions and decisions based on prior experiences and judgments.

Additionally, the brain uses the process of emotional tagging to helps us determine whether or not to pay attention to something or someone. This process elicits and extracts any emotional information attached to the experiences and thoughts stored in our memories. This emotional information gives us clues on the type of actions we should be considering and contemplating. Unfortunately, when stress overloads and overburdens the regions of the brain responsible for controlling emotions and emotional reactions, the emotional tagging process is interfered with and inhibited.

When either of these two processes is impeded or obstructed, *mind full* individuals turn into slow and incompetent decision makers. The three main ways these processes are hindered and constrained are from:

:

Inappropriate self-interest — which makes us more willing and likely to perceive the patterns we want to see.

Distorting emotional attachments — the bonds we form with people, places, and things can affect the judgments we form and the actions we are most likely to take.

Misleading memories — which cause us to overlook or undervalue critical differentiating factors that make the current circumstances not as analogous, relevant, and comparable to previous situations as our memories are leading us to believe.

Based on the way our brains work using pattern recognition and emotional tagging processes, it is not easy for *mind full* individuals to spot and prevent themselves from making errors in judgment and poor decisions. This is why it is crucial to switch from *mind full* to *mindful* mode in order to make better decisions — based on better thinking — that result in better outcomes.

Another result of being in *mind full* mode is the inability to control thoughts.

Having restless, uncontrollable, unpredictable, and fluctuating thoughts running through the brain is often called "monkey brain." These thought patterns can often hold us hostage, causing an unwillingness to take action or make decisions accompanied by fear, anxiety, stress, and negativity.

Why are we so susceptible to monkey brain? It comes from the constant, almost ceaseless barrage of decisions to make, risks to weigh, opportunities to scrutinize, interpersonal issues to deal with, and various other challenges. When the brain does not get a break from handling these never-ending issues, it gets overwhelmed and besieged with a desire to enforce its own cognitive break. Monkey mind is the brain's way of fighting back when overworked and overstimulated.

Mindfulness is an excellent way to re-take control over monkey brain. A few quiet moments of calm introspection, or simply giving the brain a break by focusing on something peaceful and soothing, helps quiet monkey brain activity and thoughts. This will defuse the rhetoric cascading around your head and let you regain concentration and focus on what you should be attending to in the present moment.

Our lives operate based on our thinking. Each of us makes decisions and takes action as a result of our respective thinking processes. Hence — and this is very important in the information overload world in which all of us live and operate — it is not just *what* you think, but *how* you think that makes a difference in the outcomes you generate.

As you will see in the next chapter, stress is a significant factor impacting the decision-making process, particularly when you are operating in *mind full* mode.

CHAPTER 3

Stress Leads to Poor Thinking and Bad Decisions

Stress is a major obstacle in life. A recent survey from the American Psychological Association (APA) states that nearly 50% of Americans are kept awake at night due to stress. (And this was before the 2020 coronavirus pandemic!)

Plus, numerous studies have shown that cumulative and chronic stress are each linked to a higher risk of both heart attack and stroke.

The APA has identified Generation X (those born between 1965 and 1979) as the most stressed generation in the United States. I suspect the Millennials will soon surpass them. And this will be troublesome, for the Millennials generation is now in the throes of parenthood, and one thing is certain — stressed parents create stressed out children. We might rightly call today's cadre of children and teenagers Generation Stressed Out.

As Dr. Kristen Race wrote in *Psychology Today* (April 2018), "Stress is both debilitating and highly contagious, so it makes perfect sense that a generation of stressed-out parents is raising a generation of stressed-out kids."

Another stress factor is impatience. When you are impatient, you feel rushed, stressed, and unhappy. Your stress hormone levels rise, which in turn can lead to a panic or anxiety attack. Impatience can also lead to snap judgments and decisions. People who lack patience are unable to delay gratification, which in turn fills them with frustration.

On the other hand, patience puts you in direct control of yourself. Patience, which can readily be brought on by the mindfulness techniques on pages 145-150, gives you the ability to remain calm and collected in the face of adversity, distress, and disappointment. It is the antidote to the stress caused by our 24/7, hectic, non-stop, fast-paced way of living.

Stress in the Workplace

Congratulations American workers, employees, and leaders!

According to an annual survey by the American Psychological Association, Americans have set a new record for stress and anxiety (again, pre-pandemic). The most commonly shared explanation for these high levels of stress in the U.S. is the nation's extreme political polarization. Other factors include uncertainty about health care, medical bills, the cost of medication, the future of the nation, money, work, social divisiveness, the economy, unemployment, low wages, climate change, environmental issues, and trust in government.

In my work with leaders in Europe, Asia, Australia, and Latin American, I hear and see evidence of the same increased stress levels. They also list many of the same causes (minus health care and medical expenses in Australia, Canada, and Europe — where national systems of public health care prevail). So high levels of stress are not just an American condition.

In fact, *The Guardian* newspaper reported that workplace stress costs U.K. businesses some £6.5B per year. While this pales to the estimated $500B per annum that workplace stress costs employers in the U.S., there is no doubt that workplace stress has a significant impact on profitability and productivity across the world. In many ways, we are all suffering the symptoms of the epidemic of stress sweeping the world today.

According to the American Institute of Stress (AIS) website, "Numerous studies show that job stress is far and away the major source of stress for American adults and that it has escalated precariously over the past few decades."

As a result, people must not only handle their own personal stress levels, but they also need to monitor and deal with the stress levels of their co-workers. Here are some of the statistics from the AIS website showing how stressful today's workplaces are:

- 40% of workers reported their jobs as very or extremely stressful.
- 25% view their jobs as the number one stressor in their lives.
- 29% of workers felt quite a bit or extremely stressed at work.
- Job stress is more strongly associated with health complaints than financial or family problems.
- Nearly half of workers say they need help in learning how to manage stress, and 42% say their coworkers need such help.
- 14% of workers had felt like striking a coworker in the past year but did not.
- 25% have felt like screaming or shouting because of job stress.

- 10% are concerned about an individual at work they fear could become violent.
- 18% had experienced some sort of threat or verbal intimidation in the past year.
- 14% said they worked where machinery or equipment was damaged because of workplace rage.
- 19% had quit a previous position because of job stress.
- Almost 25% had been driven to tears because of workplace stress.

No wonder the American Psychological Association identified Generation X as the most stressed generation in America! They now form the bulk of the workforce, and thus are experiencing the kinds of workplace stress cited by AIS in the above statistics.

We all know that being in close proximity to someone who is in a foul mood can result in our own disposition souring. And leaders know all too well that their own negative dispositions and moods can, directly and indirectly, impact direct reports, team members, and colleagues. We are now learning that the same may be true for stress.

A study published in *Nature Neuroscience* showed that stress may be contagious and that even the effect of stress on the brain may be transferable to others. While this study was conducted on mice, what is initially proven in mice is often later confirmed in human beings.

In this study, mice were exposed to mild stress and then returned to their partners. The most remarkable result of this experiment was that the neurons in the mice not exposed to the stress became altered in the exact same way as their stress exposed partners.

Again, while this has not been scientifically proven in humans, we would all be well advised to use mindfulness techniques to control and reduce our own stress levels, rather than exposing our stressful states to others in the workplace.

Impact of Stress

As athletes are well aware, peak performance can be activated through moderate and short-term periods of stress. Thus, feeling slightly nervous and anxious about an important presentation or meeting can actually prompt better performance. Hence, as long as stress is not experienced for lengthy periods, it is generally harmless and can even be beneficial.

The same is not true for prolonged periods of stress or moments when stress levels are at extremely elevated levels. In addition to increasing the risk of heart disease, depression, hypertension, and obesity, this kind of stress decreases cognitive performance. This impact can affect memory recall and cause disruptions to a person's decision-making processes.

When we are exposed to long periods of stress (as most of us are today), increased levels of glucose and fatty acids in our blood significantly raise the risk of cardiovascular disease and diabetes. A study at University College London concluded that stress also raises cholesterol levels, another known factor that increases the risk of cardiovascular disease.

In fact, stress can have significant adverse effects on our bodies, minds, emotions, and behavior as well. Here is a short summary of some of the major negative impacts of stress:

Body
Fatigue and general tiredness

Headaches

Frequent infections

Muscle tightness

Breathing difficulties

Skin irritations

Involuntary muscle twitching

Mind
Increased periods of worry

Increased procrastination

Impaired judgment

Reduced self-control

Inability to make decisions

Making hasty decisions without forethought and contemplation

Nightmares and bad dreams

Muddled, foggy thinking

Lack of clarity

Inability to focus or concentrate

Emotions
Apathy

Irritability

Quick to anger

Depression

Negativity

Moodiness

Alienation and social withdrawal

Apprehension, nervousness

Behavior
Loss of appetite or binge eating

Decreased libido

Increased alcohol consumption, alcohol abuse

Sleep difficulties, including insomnia

More frequent smoking

Accident prone, carelessness

The effects of constant and chronic stress are well known. In his book *The Happiness Handbook*, Dr. David Lee cites Robert Sapolsky, a professor of biological sciences and an authority on stress at Stanford University, in explaining how stress impacts our bodies. "In fight-or-flight mode, your body turns off all the long-term building and repair projects," explains Sapolsky. "Constant high levels of cortisol take your body's eye off the ball. Memory and accuracy are both impaired. Patrols for invaders aren't sent out, you tire more easily, you become depressed and reproduction gets downgraded."

Interestingly, our bodies are so wired and attuned to stress, because it is our internal mechanism for keeping us safe, that our systems do not differentiate between real and imagined stress triggers. That is why when we worry about a future event, or ruminate excessively about something from the past, our bodies produce the same hormones like adrenal cortisol that they would if we were facing a physical threat such as a mugging scenario.

Thus, even though no physical or other real-life stress-inducing factors are present, your body will produce these hormones when you are feeling anxious or fearful about a decision you need to make or an action you need to take. The secretion of these "fight or flight" hormones into your blood in turn triggers secretions in the brain not conducive to clear-headed thinking, judgment, and decision making.

Inflammation is the defensive response of the body's immune system to threats such as an infection or a strained muscle. Scientists now know that stress can also cause an increase of inflammation within the body, much like an infection or a turned ankle. This inflammatory response to stress in the body also impacts how the brain functions cognitively and how it regulates emotional response.

There are other ways that stress impacts our bodies, many of which are warning signs of intense or prolonged periods of stress. These include bad breath, tender or bleeding gums, sore and tense muscles, heavy breathing through the mouth, and an appetite that is never fully satisfied. Weirdly, stress can also make you not want to eat at all (we each react to stress in our own ways). Similarly, both diarrhea and constipation can result from stress.

In addition, having adrenal cortisol coursing through the body in response to stress depresses the immune system. This can lead to feelings of being burnt out and exhausted, which in turn leads to further stress. To say the least, stress is a very nasty cycle impacting our bodies, brains, emotions, and thoughts.

Stress also tends to negatively impact our sleep cycles. One might think that feeling burned out and exhausted would result in a greater propensity for sleep. And sometimes it does, for a few days. Unfortunately, this type of sleep often leaves us more lethargic and de-energized than before, which again induces more stress. As above, it is a vicious cycle.

The most common impact of stress on quality sleep is insomnia, a condition that includes trouble getting to sleep and/or staying asleep. Stress can hinder your ability to wind down and get to sleep. It can also cause a series of racing thoughts that prevents your mind from shutting down and granting you the deep sleep you so rightly deserve. The connection between sleep and stress is a complicated and highly integrated relationship.

Prolonged daily stress, and the resultant production and accumulation of adrenal cortisol in your body, also impacts your digestion system and metabolism, including your body's ability to absorb nutrients. Additionally, stress can cause your esophagus to go into spasm, increase stomach acid making you feel nauseous, affect the contractions of your digestive system, and even decrease the secretions needed for proper digestion.

The physical effects of stress include weight change, elevated blood pressure, indigestion, and inflammation. And adrenal fatigue, from too many stress-fighting hormones rushing through your system, is a cause of the mental effects of stress such as moodiness, irritability, and brain fog.

Interestingly, some of the so-called productivity tools we bring into our lives actually increase our stress levels instead of decreasing them. Smartphones are just one great example. The constant availability to check email and social media reduces our opportunities to switch off and give our brains a break.

Additionally, all the buzzes, beeps, chimes, and other electronic noise notifications jolt our stress hormones into action, similar to more dire fight-or-flight situations. Notice your reactions the next time your smartphone tells you there is something "important" for you to see. Chances are, if you pause long enough to notice instead of instinctively reaching for your mobile device, you will likely detect a slight change in your breathing pattern, a quicker heartbeat, muscles contracting or tightening, a rumble of unease in the gastrointestinal area, or even some slight perspiration forming in your palms or above your eyes.

Are any of these physical disturbances, albeit as slight as they may be, worth the constant whirl of notifications? And, while small in nature, what will be the cumulative effect of these physical reactions over time on your overall health and wellbeing? I can guarantee you, it will not be positive.

There is simply no need to live a life constantly tethered to a mobile device. At a minimum, turn off those social media notifications. When possible — and it is definitely possible — switch your mobile devices to airplane mode for an hour or two a day. You will be amazed at how refreshed and calm you feel during these mobile device sabbatical periods.

In an article in the *Australian Financial Review* (March 11, 2018), endocrinologist Robert Lustig of the University of California San Francisco writes, "Notifications from our phones are training our brains to be in a nearly constant state of stress and fear by establishing a stress-fear memory pathway. And such a state means that the prefrontal cortex, the part of our brains that normally deals with some of our highest-order cognitive functioning, goes completely haywire, and basically shuts down."

Impact of Stress on Your Brain

It is obvious that too much stress is bad for overall health, and this includes the overall health of the brain. A recent study conducted at Yale University found that prolonged stress causes degeneration in the area of the brain responsible for self-control. That is why drug use, alcohol abuse, and binge eating sends overly stressed people down the slippery slope of self-destruction. Extreme and continuous periods of stress disable the ability to exercise self-control overeating habits, drug abuse, and excessive alcohol intake.

There is a considerable increase in cognitive stress than ever before, mostly as a result of information overload combined with an ever-increasing array of distractions and interruptions. We all need to take a collective deep breath, pause, and regain control of our reactionary minds.

An article in the *Harvard Business Review* (Feb 2009) indicates the brain is wired to be more reactionary under stress. This flight-or-flight wiring results in stressed-out people falling prey to binary choice decision making, which limits the options they take into consideration.

As Ron Carucci writes in a subsequent *Harvard Business Review* (August 2017) article, "In tough moments, we reach for premature conclusions rather than opening ourselves to more and better options."

Carucci goes on to conclude that, "Faced with less familiar conditions for which our tried-and-true approaches won't work, we reflexively counter our natural anxiety by narrowing and simplifying our options. Unfortunately, the attempt to improve certainty on the uncertain tends to oversimplify things to a black-and-white, all-or-nothing extreme."

If a stress experience is too overwhelming for the usual memory retrieval and processing of the situation, our brains instinctively shift to survival mode. In survival mode, memories and previous response patterns developed in reaction to prior stressful experiences can derail our emotional and cognitive responses.

This often leads to behaviors, actions, and verbal outbursts which do not fit the circumstances and which do not help to alleviate the situation. Our reactionary actions, behaviors, and words often make the situation worse, thus increasing the stress levels for all involved.

Stress causes a flood of neurohormones to rush to the prefrontal cortex. These neurohormones impair the processing function of the prefrontal cortex, while simultaneously strengthening the emotional responses generated by the amygdala. This also causes both the amygdala and the prefrontal cortex to change structurally.

At the cellular level, dendrites are the branches of nerve cells that receive electrochemical stimulation from nearby neurons. The rushing in of neurohormones created from stress stimuli causes atrophy in the dendrites of the prefrontal cortex and extension of the dendrites found in the amygdala. This leads to fewer neurons firing in the thinking brain (prefrontal cortex) and more neurons firing off in the emotional brain (amygdala).

As a result, emotions override cognitive thinking, and we all know how well that typically works out. And, of course, poorly modulated emotional responses not only fail to resolve most stressful situations, they also tend to lead to more stress and more impaired cognitive functioning.

Not all stress, of course, is bad. Moderate and intermittent levels of stress produce adrenalin, a chemical that improves short-term performance and increases alertness.

In addition, research at the University of California Berkeley found that the onset of stress actually prompts the brain to grow new cells responsible for memory. Unfortunately, this effect is only witnessed when stress is intermittent. When such stress continues beyond a few months into a protracted state, the brain's ability to develop new brain cells is quickly suppressed.

How the Brain and Body Communicate During Stress

Research from the field of neuroscience continues to provide new evidence and clues on what happens in the brain during moments of threats and stress.

Functionally, the amygdala is the emotional control center of the brain, triggering and regulating the fight-flight-freeze response. Fortunately, especially when threats are perceived, the amygdala responds automatically and immediately. Unfortunately, however, it can also respond irrationally.

When faced with a threatening situation (real or imagined), the amygdala releases a rush of stress hormones (mostly adrenal cortisol) that floods the body before the prefrontal lobe (the regulating executive function control center of the brain) can mediate this impulse reaction. As a result, the survival instinct of the amygdala reacts before the rational functions within the brain have time to think through the situation logically.

Any strong emotion, such as anxiety, joy, anger, fear, and worry, sets off the amygdala and impairs the working memory of the prefrontal cortex. In essence, the power of emotions overwhelms rationality. This is why we cannot think straight or rationally when we are emotionally excited, upset, agitated, or stressed.

An easy way of grasping what is happening within the brain, and between your brain and your body, during times of increased stress is to think of the brain as having four core functions. These core functions are the alarm and fear center (amygdala), the thinking center (prefrontal cortex), the filing center (working and recall memory), and the emotional regulation center (anterior cingulate cortex).

The thinking center of the prefrontal cortex is located near the top of the head, behind the forehead. It is responsible for a range of functions and abilities, including rational thoughts, problem solving, planning, empathy, self-awareness, and individual personality. When this section of the brain is in charge, we are able to think clearly, be aware of ourselves and others, and make good, decisive decisions.

Near the prefrontal cortex, but located deeper inside the brain, is the anterior cingulate cortex (ACC). This section has major (but not full) responsibility for regulating emotions. Ideally, it will have a close working relationship with the prefrontal cortex areas, but this is not always the case.

When the ACC region is strong, a person is better able to manage and control difficult emotions and thoughts without being overwhelmed and incapacitated by them. When functioning effectively, the ACC helps us manage our emotions so that we do not do or say things we will later regret.

The amygdala is a smallish structure located deep inside the brain that serves as our fear and alarm center. Because of its importance for our survival, this subcortical area is outside our conscious awareness or control. Its primary function is to receive all incoming information from our five senses (seeing, hearing, smelling, touching, and tasting) and assess this information on one solitary criterion: Is this a threat?

If the amygdala determines that a threat is present, it produces fear in us. The higher the perceived level of danger from the threat, the higher the fear level. Simultaneously, it also sends signals to the body to produce a fight, flight, or freeze response. All this is done unconsciously and automatically without our cognitive control.

Of course, communication between our brains and our bodies is not a one-way street. Our bodies are constantly communicating stimuli to our brains, as well as continuously providing life-nourishing blood and oxygen flow. Here again, some of this body to brain communication is automated and subconsciously conducted without our cognitive involvement.

For instance, the average respiratory rate for adults is 12-16 breaths per minute. However, this can increase to 20 or more breaths per minute when a person is panicked or highly stressed. The body's innate response to fear and stress through faster breathing impacts brain functions and likely results in faster response times to dangerous or stressful stimuli.

While this is great when a life-threatening or serious injury threat appears (i.e., move fast a fire is approaching), it backfires on us in less dangerous scenarios. If the stress is causing an emotional outburst that the ACC cannot control, faster breathing simply hastens this harmful reaction. The increased oxygen flow to the brain is merely speeding up the emotional hijacking and resultant undesirable behavioral response.

This is why rhythmic breathing (see pages 126-130) is crucial for helping the ACC regain emotional control and to enable the prefrontal cortex to take back overall response control from the amygdala. Doing so leads to better decisions and more appropriate emotions and actions.

When stress hits and our rational coping mechanisms are overwhelmed, the alarm center (amygdala) takes over from the thinking center (prefrontal cortex). This moves us from normal mode into survival mode, due to the brain's perceived presence of fearful stimuli.

The placement of the limbic brain, which comes before the prefrontal cortex brain region, means that our limbic system, or our feelings system, reacts before anything else. The vagus nerve is at the heart of the limbic system and connects the brain physically to the body. The vagus nerve travels from the back of the brain through all of the body's organs and systems.

The vagus nerve communicates to the brain how we are feeling. Likewise, the feelings in various parts of the body contain information that is sent to the brain via the vagus nerve. Similarly, what we are thinking about will be delivered throughout the body by the vagus nerve.

This is why we may feel nervous about making a decision. In such a case, either the unease about the decision is causing negative feelings in the body to be communicated to the brain, or thoughts of doubts and any lack of confidence in the decision are being communicated to the body, thereby causing nervousness or anxiety to surface.

The vagus nerve signals any disconnect between mind and body through various physical sensations, including dryness in the throat, palpitations in the heart beat, and queasiness in the gastrointestinal region.

The intricate interconnectivity between the mind and body is multidimensional. Yet it is all too forgotten, particularly in the busyness of today's world. We typically believe that we are strictly rational with our thinking, but what we are feeling is often a more significant driver and determinant of both our decisions and actions.

Impact of Stress on Decision Making

Feeling stressed changes how people weigh risks and rewards during the decision-making process.

Surprisingly, when under stress, people actually focus more on the way outcomes could turn out right. When under stress, the natural tendency is to pay more considerable attention to positive information, while discounting negative information, according to research published in *Current Directions in Psychological Science*.

This means when people under stress are making a difficult decision, they will tend to pay more attention to the upsides of the alternatives under consideration and less attention to the downsides. The disastrous decision-making around the choice to launch the space shuttle *Challenger* is an unfortunate example of wrongfully paying too much attention to the upsides and not enough on the contradicting downsides information.

Research has also shown that stress increases the differences in how men and women think about and evaluate risk. When men are under stress, they have an increased tendency and willingness to take risks. When women are under stress, they tend to get more conservative about risk.

This, of course, is a generalization, and even though there is scientific evidence to support this conclusion, it is critically important to remember that each of us has individual tendencies, tolerances, and preferences that may or may not be in line with stereotypical gender generalizations.

Other research has shown that stress from disruptions can significantly impact decision making. Participants scored much lower on a memory exercise when disruptions and interruptions occurred. In a 2009 article in *Psychological Science*, the authors of this study also noted that when under stress while needing to make a decision, we are "more likely to bear in mind things that have been rewarding and to overlook information predicting negative outcomes." This conclusion is in agreement with the study referenced above about the tendency to focus on upsides, instead of downsides, when making decisions under stress.

Also, people under stress are more likely to make intuitive and quick decisions without really thinking through the problem or task. This is because our brains are wired to be reactionary, not analytical, under stress.

Additionally, a common propensity under stress is to resort to decision making based on binary choices. Thus, people under stress tend to limit the options available to them to just two alternatives, usually in an attempt to arrive at a faster decision. Unfortunately, this not only prevents more and often better options from being considered, but this can also result in premature conclusions based on only a subset of all available facts and information.

Most of us fall somewhere in between the two extremes of the "just trust your gut" decision maker and the "paralysis by analysis" let's analyze everything again and again decision maker. We tend to move along this continuum reasonably easily, depending on the difficulty and perceived risks of a particular decision and our ow proclivities.

However, it is essential to know ourselves, our preferences, and our default mode when it comes to decision making. This is because, when under stress, we are most likely to fall into our default mode and preferred decision-making style, no matter how easy or difficult a decision may be. This is why stress causes some people to freeze and incapacitates their decision-making capabilities, even for the easiest and most routine of decisions.

As mentioned in the previous chapter, we rely on a pair of hardwired processes for decision making. Using pattern recognition, our brains assess what appears to be going on. We then react to this information, or ignore it, due to the emotional tags stored in our memories. While usually highly reliable, these two processes can and do let us down, particularly in times of stress or tiredness.

Usually, the more stressful the circumstances, the more we need to explore a wide range of options and potential solutions. Unfortunately, while relying on past experiences may create a false sense of comfort and confidence, limiting one's options is more often than not a recipe for disaster and poor decision making.

Additionally, many poor decisions are made as a result of people feeling stressed and insecure about their jobs, their career trajectories, their own confidence, and even what others may be thinking about them.

There are tremendous pressures and expectations placed on workers in all fields, as well as students and non-working adults. As a result, it is hard not to have some stressful insecurities and occasionally feeling a lack of confidence. After all, there are so many variables every day with which to deal. So many unknowns that cannot be contemplated. So many people questioning your decisions. And so many personalities to deal with, including your own.

Of course, we all have insecurities at times, thinking that we are not good enough or that we are likely to fail on a particular assignment or task. Insecurities can be quite overwhelming at times, especially given the fear that a failure might have an adverse impact on employment, social status, or future financial security. Here is what often drives such stressful fears of failure and insecurities:

- Need for constant validation and approval.
- Ruminating and dwelling on past criticisms.
- Lack of trust in others, particularly peers and superiors at work or family members and friends outside work.
- Inability to accept self-imperfections and one's own mistakes, and a history of blaming mistakes and errors on outside, uncontrollable factors.

- Falsely comparing one's self with those perceived to be more successful.

Another decision-making peril caused by stress is the tendency for leaders, particularly new supervisors and mid-level leaders, to start (or increase) micromanaging. This is also noticeable with small business owners and entrepreneurs in new start-up ventures. If this happens frequently, it can have significant long-term negative consequences for their teams, as micromanaging is cited as one of the most common reasons why employees quit. No one likes to be micromanaged by their leader.

As you will read in the next chapter, mindfulness is a proven, skillful method for stress reduction and all of the many associated ills and problems that result from accumulated stress. Additionally, stress reduction through mindfulness practices is a proven performance advantage that comes with the side benefits of greater happiness, health, and wellbeing.

Impact of Emotional Stress on Decision Making

Emotions are a central part of our lives, dictating and influencing our thoughts, desires, intentions, actions, and decisions. Emotions also influence our attitudes, perspectives, and our judgments.

Emotions are easily triggered by worry. Humans, unfortunately, are wired to worry. Our brains are continually imagining futures we hope will meet our needs and desires. That would be fine. But our brains also spend too much time generating thoughts about the possible obstacles, hurdles, and bumps that might block us from attaining our goals, objectives, hopes, and dreams.

Worry causes emotional stress, which often results in sleepless nights, preoccupation with negative thoughts or fears, tension, and physical ailments. These distract us from the very important tasks and projects that should be the center of our attention.

Our brains are wired to react. It is how our brains have evolved, from primeval times when faster reactions meant longer lives and potentially more progeny. Fast reactions meant survival, plain and simple.

Unfortunately, this wiring favors the amygdala over the prefrontal cortex. The result is that decision making can be undesirably affected by the overreacting amygdala hijacking the brain's ability to produce rational and complex thinking. Fortunately, such hijacks can be mitigated with practice and persistence.

Our emotional state in any given moment influences what we see and perceive, according to a study published in *Psychological Science*. What we see is not a direct reflection of the world, but rather a mental representation of the world that is induced by our emotional experiences.

"We do not passively detect information in the world and then react to it — we construct our perceptions of the world as the architects of our own experience. Our affective feelings are a critical determinant of the experience we create," the researchers from the University of California San Francisco reported. "That is, we do not come to know the world through only our external senses — we see the world differently when we feel pleasant or unpleasant."

The gist of this is to understand that your varying moods will influence your perceptions and valuations of the people you are dealing with, as well as the information, suggestions, opinions, and recommendations you are receiving from them.

Emotions are powerful. They dictate your mood and, if left unchecked, compel you to react instead of responding to situations, events, and people. Gaining control over your emotions will enable you to become mentally stronger and empower you to respond to situations, events, and people instead of automatically and emotionally reacting to them.

A straightforward way to gain control over your emotions is to hit the pause button. This provides time for you to access the frontal lobes of your brain, which drives reasoning, problem solving, and perspective.

This may sound too simple, but as Dr. Amelia Aldao, a therapist, recommends, "wait 60 seconds before doing anything to gain better control of our emotions."

Dr. Aldao, who has spent over a decade studying how people can better control their emotions, explains: "That's it; simple as that. Just wait. Hit the pause button. Don't do anything. In particular, don't follow what the emotion is telling you to do. Don't send that angry text. Don't decline the invitation to present at work, don't tell your potential date you're too busy this week, don't send that passive-aggressive email to your boss. Just don't."

Pausing before reflexively acting, so that you can respond instead of reacting, is one of the hardest things for people to do. This is because our natural inclination is to allow our emotions to get the best of us. We give in to our feelings. Too easily. And that is a behavior that needs to change if we want to make better decisions and create better outcomes.

Fortunately, regulating one's emotions is a skill and, like any skill, can be learned, practiced, enhanced, and ingrained through effort, patience, and persistence. Regulating, or managing, your emotions does not mean suppressing them. Especially if they are intensively and deeply felt emotions. Sure, if something is just a little upsetting, you can choose to ignore such a feeling and move on. But if you attempt to suppress strongly felt emotions on the pretense that you do not want to offend somebody, then you are the one most likely to end up hurt and wounded.

Unaddressed negative emotions do not get solved by themselves. The saying that "time heals all wounds" is definitely not true. Time may heal some wounds. But in most instances, the passage of the time merely takes the edge and sharpness off acute pain. In fact, suppressed feelings and emotions usually lead to negative coping strategies, such as excessive food intake, alcohol, or drugs. None of these are good decision-making or rational thinking strategies. All three of them lead to more emotional stress in one's life.

While it is important to recognize and acknowledge your feelings and emotions, it is more important to recognize, acknowledge, and deeply understand that your feelings and emotions do not have to control you.

When your emotions get you down, especially when you need a clear head for making decisions or complex thinking, the three best things you can do are:

1. Label your emotions. Labeling how you are feeling can take a lot of the heat and hurt out of the emotion. Most important, labeling your emotions helps you to pause and consider how these feelings may be affecting your decisions and thinking at that moment.

2. Reframe your thoughts. Pause and consider the emotional filter through which you are viewing a situation, event, or person. If you are in a good mood, is this causing you to misinterpret information too positively? If you are in a negative emotional state, is this causing you to misinterpret information too negatively? An email with positive feedback from your boss

does not necessarily translate into a job promotion or a raise. Likewise, an email of criticism from your boss does not necessarily mean you are on the road to being fired.

Reframing your thoughts means taking the judgment out of them and developing a more realistic point of view.

3. Engage in a mood booster when in a negative emotional state. Take a walk outside. Occupy yourself with a few moments of mindfulness (see chapters 8 and 9 for a range of mindfulness techniques). Call a friend, family member, or even a colleague to talk about something pleasant (but no complaining!).

Another interesting revelation from recent research is that when we are angry, we apparently believe we are smarter than everyone else around us. This tendency to think that everyone is automatically dumber than ourselves when we are furious and feverishly angry was discovered in 2018 in a research study published in the journal *Intelligence*. The researchers studied people with trait anger.

The Encyclopedia of Behavioral Medicine defines trait anger as a "dispositional characteristic where one experiences frequent anger, with varying intensity and is often accompanied by related negative emotions such as envy, resentment, hate, and disgust."

People afflicted with trait anger are more likely to be described as having a fiery personality characterized by hot-temperateness and are also more likely to actually get angry. They are also more likely to display signs of narcissism — believing their world revolves around them — and go into episodes of rage when it does not.

Those with trait anger are more likely to wrongly think they are far more intelligent than the people around them, and thus less likely to consider the thoughts and ideas of others when making decisions. It is also harder to rationally argue with people who have trait anger as tend to react angrily to any comments or suggestions that oppose their views.

One of the best ways to prevent stress, especially emotional stress, from impacting your decision making and thinking is to regularly stop and ask yourself this one simple question:

In what situations and interpersonal interactions do I regularly find my emotions and reactions working against me and my best interests?

Truly understanding the answer to this question — and then taking proactive steps to prevent emotional hijacking in such situations and interactions — is a sure-fire route to better decisions, better thinking, and better outcomes.

The next chapter will provide ideas and techniques for reducing work-related and personal stress, as well as ways to cope and handle general emotional stress and anxiety.

CHAPTER 4

Reducing Stress for Better Decisions and Better Outcomes

If the previous chapter did not convince you to significantly reduce stress in your life, I do not know what will.

Neuroscience research is now revealing that mindfulness practices and meditation can train the brain to be less reactive to emotional swings. These techniques can also help prevent the wrong brain modules from hijacking control of our thinking and decisions.

In his book *Altered Traits: Science Reveals How Meditation Changes Your Mind, Brain, and Body*, Daniel Goleman describes a study conducted with Buddhist monks:

> *The meditators' brains were scanned while they saw disturbing images of people suffering, like burn victims. The seasoned practitioners' brains revealed a lowered level of reactivity in the amygdala; they were more immune to emotional hijacking. The reason: their brains had stronger operative connectivity between the prefrontal cortex, which manages reactivity, and the amygdala, which triggers such reactions. As neuroscientists know, the stronger this particular link*

in the brain, the less a person will be hijacked by emotional downs and ups of all sorts.

When you are better able to cope with and control your feelings, rather than just reacting instinctively to them, the greater will be your ability to remain calm and reject an emotional hijacking. And, of course, the less you are hijacked by emotional swings, the better decisions you will make. This is why the first decision to make is the decision to pause and become determined to respond, rather than react.

The importance of maintaining control over the interactions between emotions and the brain has long been a secret of success for those in high-pressure careers, from ancient Samurai warriors to astronauts and Navy SEALs. We are now at a time when this knowledge can be applied to decision making for all of us, in both our professional and personal lives.

Stress is an enemy of short-term working memory, which lets you briefly hold and manipulate information in your brain. In military personnel, this skill is known to decline during stressful periods like combat deployment or even field training. In a University of Miami study, researchers provided eight hours of mindfulness instruction to U.S. soldiers over a month during their pre-deployment training. These researchers tested the soldiers' short-term memory before and after the intervention.

In the soldiers who completed a mindfulness program that emphasized in-class exercises, researchers detected no deterioration in working memory. In a second group, soldiers who took a lecture-focused mindfulness course, memory scores dipped slightly. In the third group, the soldiers who got no mindfulness training at all showed the highest slippage in working memory scores.

By bolstering cognitive resilience, the researchers say, mindfulness may help prevent errors during combat. Civilians in high-stress, high-performance situations could very well reap similar benefits.

There are many ways to reduce stress in your life:

1. Limit (or eliminate) watching and listening to the news, particularly cable television news shows. You can still stay informed, particularly if you substitute broadcast news with an app that allows you to view a wide range of media articles and video clips.

    When news is continuously presented in dramatic, news-breaking fashion — as it is on all the cable television broadcasts — it creates anxiety, fear, anger, and stress.

2. Practice mindfulness by focusing only on what is happening in the present moment. Bring forth self-awareness, compassion, and nonjudgmental thinking through the mindfulness techniques described in chapters 8 and 9. Respond with knowledge, insight, and forethought to the present moment rather than reacting in ways that create more stress or result in regrettable emotional outbursts or inappropriate action.

3. Focus on what you can control. You are unlikely to have absolute control over everything in your professional or personal life. Work and live as best you can within the parameters given.

4. Seek support, but do not unilaterally dump your problems, woes, and concerns on others. Support is best when it is a two-way street. Share your feelings and thoughts with like-minded people who can help you feel understood and supported. This alone will help to reduce the stress you are feeling. Be careful not to turn these conversations into office politics and back-stabbing gossip sessions.

Other effective stress coping strategies are:

- Taking long, deep breaths.
- Short meditation sessions of three to five minutes.
- Maintaining one's sense of humor.
- Walking outside (sunshine and fresh air are two of nature's top stress antidotes).
- Reframing thoughts or fears into challenges to be overcome or dealt with to the best of your ability.
- Any of the mindfulness techniques found in chapters 8 and 9.

And, there is also my personal favorite: eat moderate amounts of dark chocolate. People who eat more dark chocolate are less stressed, according to two recent scientific studies. These studies report that dark chocolate, with at least 70% concentration of cocoa, can have positive effects on stress, inflammation, memory, mood, and even the immune system.

Other reported benefits include enhanced neuroplasticity, which is the brain's ability to adjust and create new neuronal connections as we encounter, learn, and adapt to new things and experiences. There is more on the benefits of moderate dark chocolate consumption near the end of this chapter.

Purposeful Breathing

This takes us back to using purposeful breathing to regain control when stress stimuli appear and multiply. Practicing purposeful breathing (see chapter 8) daily, even for just three to five minutes at a time, can help to de-stress your life.

Practicing purposeful breathing calms the stress responses emanating from the brain during moments of elevated stress. Additionally, the more you practice purposeful breathing at times when you are not under stress, the better you will become at using this technique as a de-stressing and calm-inducing tool when it is most needed.

Regular purposeful breathing practice strengthens the neural pathways in the anterior cingulate cortex (ACC) region of the brain. As noted previously, this is the area of the brain that helps us maintain focus and attention, think clearly when we are upset, and prompts emotional intelligence to surface in our interactions with others. Keeping this part of the brain healthy and strong does wonders for how we engage with the people around us and for how we can be more intentional and stress-reducing in our actions, behaviors, and thoughts.

Diaphragmatic breathing (or what I call purposeful breathing — see chapter 8) instantly stimulates the vagus nerve and lowers the stress responses associated with the fight-flight-freeze mechanisms in the body. Stimulating the vagus nerve through deep, purposeful breathing not only reduces stress, but it also lowers anxiety, anger, and inflammation by activating the relaxation response of the parasympathetic nervous system.

Let's look at some other ways to reduce stress, stay calm, and handle anxiety.

Stress Relief

Across the world, mindfulness and meditation practices are becoming less associated with only alternative lifestyles and cultures. In fact, mindfulness and meditation are increasingly becoming an essential part of the daily routines for millions and millions of people. According to TIME magazine, yoga is now practiced by 11% of Americans, and meditation is used by 9.9%.

How will this increase in personal mindfulness practices impact the workplace?

According to some, it has already begun. In a study of 85,000 adults reported in the Centers for Disease Control and Prevention journal *Preventing Chronic Disease*, "Approximately one in seven workers report engagement in some form of mindfulness-based activity, and thus individuals can bring awareness of the benefit of used practices into the workplace."

The authors of the study cited activities such as yoga and meditation as having been shown to improve employee well-being and workplace productivity. Their conclusion: "The high and increasing rates of exposure to mindfulness practices among U.S. workers is encouraging."

Additionally, the emotional intelligence service TalentSmart researched over one million people and found that 90% of top performers are skilled in remaining calm under stress.

There are numerous ways to reduce stress and its impact on your body, brain, emotions, and thinking. Some of these are useful in combating momentary stress or anxiety, while others are long-term practices that can help you manage the negative stresses in your life and aid you in making better decisions.

As in all methods for improving one's physical and mental wellbeing, it is best to consult with your physician or other certified medical practitioners before employing the techniques and methods outlined here.

Also, for the tips and ideas here that resonate with you, I encourage you to do further in-depth research on the methods, benefits, and any side effects before you start to implement them. The information below serves merely as an overview of some of the techniques and methods I have studied and utilized.

Reducing Work-Related Stress
1. Understand the normalcy of anxiety. Everyone has moments of anxiety. Unfortunately, worrying about your feelings of anxiety only serves to intensify and prolong those anxious feelings.

    Research shows that people who focus on their personal strengths and personal coping mechanisms (such as self-talk or recalling memories of past successes) in moments of anxiety can significantly decrease the strength and length of such feelings.

    On the other hand, those who designate their anxious feelings as a personal weakness and deficiency actually raise their levels of anxiety and reduce their levels of self-confidence.

2. Stay connected with peers and friends. Networking and socializing is beneficial for emotional wellbeing and quality of life. Many people isolate themselves, fearing that any inadequacies or self-doubts will be visible to others.

Interacting with peers or friends is one way to allow yourself to be vulnerable and to express your tightly held fears in a safe and trusting environment. It is also a great way to be reminded that none of us is infallible or free of errors and mistakes, which can help reduce the angst surrounding the tougher decisions we face.

3. Focus on priorities. It is very easy to allow our calendars to be filled by others, to get swamped by the minutiae of daily decision making, and to get derailed by urgent matters taking priority over important tasks. Unfortunately, crossing out 10 or 15 small decisions off your task list is unlikely to produce the significant results that come from one strategic decision made after hours of focused contemplation and analysis.

Years ago, I divided my to-do list into two separate lists, one of which has the 5-6 major priorities I am working on (such as writing this book) and the other containing my list of getting "stuff" done. That GSD list receives a significantly reduced prioritization in my life, other than when specific deadlines (like a friend's birthday or the payment due dates on bills) give them immediacy or urgency.

People who focus on priorities, and who delegate more and micromanage less, create more time for the important things in their professional and personal lives. They also carve out more time, and more mental energy, for contemplating the more significant issues and decisions confronting them.

4. Practice purposeful rhythmic breathing. As soon as your body starts to send stress signals (shortness of breath, sweaty palms, churning in the gut, overwhelming sensations in your mind), hit the pause button. Literally.

    Through purposeful breathing, you can quickly calm your nervous system and regain control over your thoughts and emotions. Purposeful breathing can be done anywhere in the office — at your desk, in a meeting surrounded by others, while walking to or from a meeting, or during a quick visit outside to enjoy some fresh air and a bit of sunshine.

    There are many techniques and methods for purposeful breathing (several of which we describe in detail in chapter 8). All of them focus on purposefully creating a rhythmic breathing pattern. None require you to take off your shoes, close your eyes (though doing so can help prevent distractions), or twisting your body into a lotus position.

    The best method is to find and practice a pattern of breathing that works best for you. Here's mine: breathe in slowly through the nose, filling the abdomen and then the lungs beyond normal inhalation; hold breath for a count of eight; exhale very slowly until the abdomen and lungs are emptied more than usual. Hold the emptiness stage for a count of eight. Repeat five to ten times as needed to regain a sense of calm and control.

Practicing such rhythmic breathing throughout the day also increases oxygen levels. When the level of oxygen reaching the brain increases, the brain responds by sending signals to the body that it can relax. Increased oxygen levels in the brain will also trigger the release of feel-good hormones (such as dopamine) that help to relieve pain and increase feelings of wellness and happiness.

5. Respond instead of reacting. There is a tremendous difference between reacting to a situation and responding. Impulsively reacting tends to add more stress, to both yourself and others. Reacting also usually results in the first thought or idea becoming a decision, which often is not the best possible solution.

    On the other hand, responding is more reflective and helps to redirect your thoughts to allow the consideration of a range of options. Responding, particularly with the phrase "let me think about that," does, in fact, help create time for adequate reflection, analysis, and contemplation. All of which will make you a better thinker and decision maker.

6. Ask the right questions instead of making an on-the-spot decision. This is not a procrastination technique unless used in the wrong way for the wrong reasons.

Reducing General Stress

1. Do not negatively judge yourself, your feelings, or your emotions. Accept how you are feeling — tired, anxious, nervous, overwhelmed, afraid, uncertain, etc. Accept the reality of how you are feeling, without judgment or self-criticism.

   Pause and reflect on the likely root causes of your feelings, again without judgment or blame (especially without blaming others or events). Own your feelings as yours. Do not try to shift ownership to someone else (i.e., she's making me feel this way). Your feelings are how you are reacting, consciously and unconsciously, to a situation, the behavior of another, or to what someone has said to you or about you. As Shakespeare wrote, "It is neither good nor bad, but thinking makes it so."

   Self-criticism for having and experiencing your feelings is nothing but an additional stress booster. Hating or chastising yourself is negative energy that stress, and many other bad feelings, feed upon. Objectively assessing what you are feeling, and the root causes of your stress, are the first steps to regaining control of your feelings and enabling rational thinking. Doing so helps prevent the emotional hijacking situations we discussed previously.

2. Write down everything that is stressing you. It takes less than ten minutes to do a mind dump of everything that is aggravating and annoying you. Writing down this list of stresses, both big and small, eliminates the urge to keep

everything bottled up in your mind (thus freeing up much-needed working memory space in your brain). It also usually results in an immediate reduction in stress levels.

3. Give yourself a break. Your body and your brain both require frequent periods of brief rest. Neither are designed to run at "Mach Two with your hair on fire" for extended periods of time. (Kudos to you if you get the gratuitous 1980s movie reference in the previous sentence.) A good rule of thumb is a five to ten-minute break every 60-75 minutes.

These breaks can be as simple as a quick walk outside to get some fresh air, or moving to a quiet place where you can do some deep breathing exercises and mild stretching of legs, torso, back, and neck muscles. When these breaks are self-satisfying, they not only re-energize your body and brain, but they also have the benefit of increasing your body's levels of dopamine.

4. Enjoy a laugh. Laughter is a powerful medicine, especially in the fight against stress. I often coach leaders to replace cable news viewing (a known stress factor) with watching a comedy show like reruns of *The Big Bang Theory*. Alternatively, 15 minutes of silliness on YouTube will lighten your stress load.

5. Make exercise an integral part of your lifestyle. When the body moves, it releases endorphins that help reduce stress levels. Exercise also

helps boost energy levels and reduce incidents of insomnia. The body holds onto stress in both the digestive tract and within tight muscles. By loosening those tight muscles, exercise and stretching effectively lower your stress load.

6. Focus on the bigger picture and the things that are most meaningful to you. Daily life provides numerous opportunities to be stressed out. But focusing on the irritations, problems, and annoyances of your day-to-day world makes these issues appear more significant than they truly are.

   Thinking about the broader context of life helps put the daily rhythm of stress into a better perspective. Yes, that flat tire you experienced on the way to work needs replacing. But at least you did not lose control of the vehicle, causing you to crash or hurt someone. In the context of what could have gone wrong for you and others from a blown tire on the highway, having to miss that "important" conference call is not so earth-shattering after all.

7. Incorporate meditation into your daily activities. We list a range of meditative practices and techniques in chapter 10.

8. Practice purposeful rhythmic breathing multiple times every day (see point four above under reducing work-related stress).

Staying Calm

My focus above mainly concerned long periods of stress. Let's now look at managing our emotions and staying calm when stress levels are momentarily escalated, often due to time-sensitive deadlines or crisis situations that suddenly appear.

In such situations, stress may actually help us perform better. No doubt you have experienced times when the pressure of deadlines forced you to concentrate better. As a result, you experienced the phenomena known as "flow," resulting in some level of peak performance.

On the other hand, instances of unexpected stress or too much pressure to handle may lead to emotional outbursts, impaired cognitive responses, and even physical ailments.

There are a few excellent techniques to help you stay calm in situations of temporary high stress, including:

- Purposefully slow down all your body movements. Slowing your motion sends signals to your body to remain calm and can prevent activation of the parasympathetic nervous system (described on pages 130-131). Additionally, slowing body movement reduces the risks of hyperventilating.

- Keeping your hand gestures at waist level, or slightly below. Doing so helps to center yourself and can also change (and slow) your breathing pattern.

- Put a hand on your upper thigh. Placing an open palm on the upper portion of your thigh mimics the calming gesture that parents and friends instinctively do to calm children. Even when you do this to yourself, it works!

Additionally, teach yourself to speak slower and in a lower tone. Speaking rapidly is a telltale sign of anxiety, nervousness, and a lack of confidence. Practicing to speak slowly builds muscle memory, enabling you to reduce anxiety in high-stress situations simply by purposefully slowing your speaking rate and lowering your tone of voice.

Here are six more methods for staying calm and controlling your emotions when stress threatens to take over a situation and hijack you either emotionally or cognitively. You will note that several of these have similarities with the techniques described above, and for a good reason — negative stress is negative stress, whether it is the short-term kind or it hangs around for lengthy periods.

1. An attitude of gratitude. Daily reminders of what you are grateful for builds a solid wall against stress. Research conducted at the University of California Davis revealed that people who spend time daily to cultivate an attitude of gratitude and thankfulness experienced improved moods, energy, and physical wellbeing. Researchers believe that such daily gratitude practices, including the keeping of a gratitude journal in some instances, lowered levels of adrenal cortisol, the hormone which is associated with increased stress.

2. Remain positive. Our brains like to wander. They also like to attach themselves to random thoughts, either negative or positive. Rather than allow our brains to decide which thoughts to focus on, we need to be proactive by focusing on stress-free and positive thoughts.

    Usually, concentrating on any positive thought will do, even recalling positive experiences or successes from your past. This comes naturally when things are going well and our moods are great. But it takes a concentrated effort to do so when negative moments and bad news comes our way.

3. Cancel the negative self-talk sessions. Spending more than a few minutes chastising yourself for a mistake, a decision that turned out wrong, or for not speaking up for yourself or your ideas in a meeting is a sure-fire way to entice more stress in your life.

    Ruminating on negative thoughts, particularly about one's self or one's actions, gives them more power to create additional stress for you to deal with. Additionally, almost all negative self-talk centers around thoughts and opinions, not facts. But continuing to discuss and reinforce these thoughts and opinions internally gives them the credence of facts to our minds.

    Clearly identifying and labeling negative self-talk as mere thoughts, and then separating them from the actual facts (i.e., you do not always make poor presentations vs. yesterday's presentation was not your best effort) will help close the cycle of negativity swimming around in your mind and help move you to a more realistic and positive outlook.

4. Focus on purposeful breathing. As discussed above (pages 73-74), pausing to focus on deep,

rhythmic breathing will help to rapidly calm both your body and your brain.

5. Reframe your perspective. It is a two-way, circular interaction. Our thoughts can increase our stress, and stress can impact our thoughts. No wonder things and situations often spiral out of control so quickly.

    While you cannot always control your circumstances, you can always control how you respond emotionally and cognitively (provided you do not grant control to stress and negative thoughts). For any stressful situation, start by putting things into perspective. Then ask yourself:

    "How can I handle this situation without over-reacting emotionally and with the full resources of my cognitive faculties?"

    Just asking this question confirms that you are purposefully taking control of your response to a given circumstance or situation. Now, list how you genuinely want to respond emotionally, either positively or neutrally. Note the phrase being used here: genuinely want to respond. It is not about how you might feel you want to react. It is about how you truly want to respond.

    Next, list what is wrong with the situation and what are the possible solutions or fixes. And remember to keep breathing, rhythmically and deeply. This too shall pass.

6. Tap into your support system. Very rarely do stressful challenges need to be handled solely and without help. Often, however, challenges become stressful because we do not have all the skills or resources to deal with them by ourselves and we are reluctant to ask for help.

This is where seeking the help, advice, and support of colleagues, peers, friends, and family members kicks in. A key to remaining calm in times of unexpected stress is knowing that help abounds in the form of your professional and personal support systems and networks. We all have weaknesses, and often the strengths and skills we need to complement our shortfalls are found within others.

Dark Chocolate Reduces Stress

Now for perhaps the best news you will find between the covers of this book, especially if you are a chocolate lover. Science has confirmed what some of us knew — and many of us hoped — all along: dark chocolate can reduce stress!

Chocolate can also reduce inflammation and improve one's mood (I think we all knew the latter, but it is nice to have it scientifically confirmed). Of course, these results also come with the caveat that chocolate should be consumed in moderation since its sugar content and high-calorie levels can impact the risks for both obesity and diabetes.

Researchers from Loma Linda University had participants eat one dark chocolate bar containing at least 70% cacao and then examined their brain waves. Gamma waves in the brains of participants showed increased activity only 30 minutes after the chocolate bars were consumed. Gamma waves signal that the nerves within the brain are working, leading to optimum learning and memory. Based on these results, it may be advisable to bring some dark chocolate to the next training program you attend.

It has been well known for many years that cacao is a primary source of flavonoids, the remarkably potent antioxidant and anti-inflammatory agents beneficial for brain and cardiovascular health. In the two studies conducted by Loma Linda University researchers, this was the first scientific proof that flavonoids also have a positive impact on cognitive memory, mood, immunity, and other beneficial effects.

In another study, researchers at Columbia University and New York University gave a large daily dose of flavanols extracted from cocoa powder to a group of participants. During the trial period, the participants reported improved memory, and tests showed enhanced blood flow to the hippocampus, the part of the brain responsible for memory formation.

Regularly eating moderate amounts of dark chocolate has also been scientifically linked to reducing blood pressure, lowering inflammation, improving sensitivity to insulin (and thus reducing the risk for Type-2 diabetes), suppressing appetite, better protection against UV radiation in sunlight, eliminating low-density cholesterol (the bad cholesterol in blood), boosting mood by stimulating the production of serotonin, and reducing stress and anxiety during pregnancy.

Perhaps one day researchers will prove that eating chocolate will improve our memories to eat more chocolate! In moderation, of course.

Handling Anxiety

Anxiety is another type of stressor that many people face. In fact, anxiety disorders are the most common mental illness in the United States, affecting over 40 million adults.

Anxiety interferes with the brain's decision-making operations, but not for the reasons you might think. It appears that people at risk for anxiety have lower activity in a region of the brain responsible for complex mental operations, according to the results of a study at Duke University.

These research findings also showed that people whose brains exhibit a higher response to threat and a lower response to reward are more at risk of developing the symptoms of anxiety and depression over time. The individual configuration of the brain has a direct impact on one's propensity to incur anxiety.

Hence, signs of anxiety and the stresses associated with anxiety impact the brain's decision-making functionality. However, these signs may also be an indicator of a reduced activity level occurring in the brain's dorsolateral prefrontal cortex, the brain's executive control center which assists in focusing attention and planning complex actions.

When anxiety strikes, even at moderate or low levels, it can seem impossible to stop the downward spirals of worries, fears, and self-doubt. In her book *How to Be Yourself: Quiet Your Inner Critic and Rise Above Social Anxiety*, Boston University clinical psychologist Ellen Hendriksen shares a mindfulness hack that can help you stay in the moment when anxiety asserts itself.

Called the 5-4-3-2-1 method, this mindfulness technique is useful any time you find yourself ruminating over particular worries or feeling anxiously overwhelmed. The technique incorporates all five senses in order to ground yourself in the present moment by having you name:

1. Five things you can see.
2. Four things you can hear.
3. Three things you can feel via the sense of touch.

4. Two things you can smell.

5. One thing you can taste.

The relationship between the quantities and each particular sense does not matter. It is only necessary that all five senses are incorporated. So feel free to mix up the above example if you want (i.e., four things you can feel and three things you can hear). Again, the most important thing is that you scroll through all five senses, using your powers of observation to get the brain to focus on 15 specific things rather than the spinning thoughts concerning your worries, concerns, fears, or anxieties.

Once you are firmly rooted in the present moment through this technique, you will be in a better position to deal more thoughtfully with those worries and concerns.

Inculcating mindfulness into your thinking patterns is a reliable way to control feelings of insecurity. By focusing on the present moment on a regular and frequent basis, you will start to:

- Nonjudgmentally accept everything about yourself.
- Move past the past.
- Avoid comparing yourself with others.
- Become more trusting of others.
- Find that the validation from yourself is the only validation that matters.

These benefits of mindfulness were best summed up by ancient Chinese philosopher Lao-Tzu: "Because one believes in oneself, one doesn't try to convince others. Because one is content with oneself, one doesn't need others' approval. Because one accepts one's self, the whole world accepts him or her."

As with most brain-related illnesses, the best cures for long-term anxiety disorders start with lifestyle changes, along with having a reliable support system of family and friends. These changes include exercising regularly, eating more healthily, creating and sticking to a sleep schedule, and incorporating mindful meditation and other relaxation techniques into a daily routine.

Of course, changing behavior can be challenging for a person living with and dealing with anxiety issues. As in all medical situations, you should check and clarify with medical professionals how these lifestyle changes will impact your particular anxiety disorder and your treatment plan.

CHAPTER 5

Mindfulness

According to the American Mindfulness Research Association, the number of papers on mindfulness published in journals rose from 10 in 2000 to almost 700 in 2016. At the same time, according to PubMed, 42,245 papers were published in 2016 on heart disease alone. So the scientific study of mindfulness is still in its infancy, but is growing rapidly.

Around 4.3 million adults in the U.S. engage in mindfulness meditation, according to an analysis of the 2012 National Health Interview Survey. Among those practicing mindfulness, the most mentioned motivations were to improve stress levels, emotional wellbeing, and general health.

Mindfulness, in its purest form, is simple and easy. You do not need a yoga mat or a sitting cushion. You do not need to learn to chant mantras, repeat phrases, or how to make particular humming sounds. And you do not need to block off significant chunks of your daily calendar to practice mindfulness.

An important point: mindfulness can be practiced within or outside meditation. Meditation is just one of the many methods available for achieving mindfulness. The same goes for yoga.

Also, you do not have to extricate yourself from reality or "go find yourself" in a darkened, quiet space. In fact, rather than trying to escape reality, mindfulness is actually a method of stepping fully into reality and becoming as close to being fully present in the moment as you possibly can.

Defining Mindfulness

Mindfulness is a state of complete (or nearly full) awareness. It is gained through the purposeful self-regulation of attention placed and maintained on the present experience, combined with a mindset that is open, curious, inquiring, and accepting. It is a sense of being psychologically and cognitively aware and accepting of the present moment.

This dimension of awareness and alertness is a methodology for clearing and refreshing (some say rebooting) the brain. The chief outcome is a slowing, even stopping, of the mind's wandering proclivities. Another key result is halting any patterns of fixedness in cognitive and emotional processing.

Mindfulness is not about thinking positively, but rather it is about learning how to think differently and realistically on a more frequent and conscious basis. Mindfulness training and practice also permanently rewire the brain, thus enabling us to change the unhelpful thinking and behavior patterns that can keep us stuck.

In the popular press, mindfulness is often discussed and defined in the context of other concepts, such as yoga, relaxation techniques, meditation, and even therapeutic strategies. And that is because mindfulness can play an important part in each of these. But mindfulness is not limited to a support role and, in fact, it is a practice unto itself.

Here are some common myths and misconceptions of mindfulness:

1. Mindfulness is more than just learning to meditate. In fact, meditation is not required for you to become more mindful and present.

2. The purpose of mindfulness is to slow down and observe thoughts without judgment, not to have zero thoughts.

3. Mindfulness is not about taking time out to relax, rest, and tune-out the world. Instead, mindfulness helps you become more attuned and aware of the world around you.

4. The ultimate goal is not to become mindful all the time, but rather to bring mindfulness into your life on a regular basis to reduce stress, control emotions, improve cognitive thinking, and make better decisions.

Mindfulness is paying attention to the present moment and to yourself in three particular ways:

1) on purpose

2) in the moment

3) without judgment

You can practice mindfulness in a variety of ways, including mindfulness of breathing, eating, bodily sensations (body scans), thoughts, emotions, communication (both listening and speaking), walking, jogging, yoga, tai chi, and many other activities. With continuous practice, you can become more mindful throughout the day, not just during dedicated mindfulness sessions.

At its core, mindfulness is a self-chosen, self-directed, and self-regulated approach to thinking and awareness that enables a person to disengage (wholly or partly) from the many stresses in life that at times can seem all-consuming. Or, in the words of global spiritual leader Thich Nhat Hanh, "I like to define mindfulness as the energy that helps us be there 100 percent. It is the energy of your true presence."

The simplest way to be mindful is to stop whatever you are doing, mentally or physically, and place your full concentration on the physical sensations of a few deep breaths as they come into and go out of your body. Doing so plants you firmly in the present moment, with a revitalized brain and a greater sense of calmness and control. As author and mindfulness teacher Sylvia Boorstein says, "Mindfulness is awake attention to what is happening inside and outside so we can respond from a place of wisdom."

The most frequently quoted definition of mindfulness comes from Jon Kabat-Zinn, the creator of the Stress Reduction Clinic and the Center for Mindfulness in Medicine, Health Care, and Society at the University of Massachusetts, "Mindfulness means paying attention in a particular way, on purpose, in the present moment, and nonjudgmentally."

In essence, mindfulness is a state of being consciously aware of the present moment and all that it entails. The "particular way" mentioned by Kabat-Zinn in my mind means fully focusing one's attention and awareness on the present moment, while calmly acknowledging and nonjudgmentally accepting the feelings, thoughts, and bodily sensations that you are having at this particular moment.

Such present moment awareness is a state of sustained awareness of — and attention to — the present moment, including being fully aware of and paying full attention to your own internal experiences, feelings, and sensations.

In short, mindfulness is a high level of alertness and open awareness that enhances focus, overall attention to the present moment, and the cognitive surfacing of options for solutions and emotional control. Achieving mindfulness involves more than just putting away your mobile phone, shutting down your computer, or turning off the television.

As Kabat-Zinn notes, "The best way to capture moments is to pay attention. This is how we cultivate mindfulness. Mindfulness means being awake. It means knowing what you are doing."

When you focus your attention on the present moment through any mindfulness technique, you immediately become more cognizant and conscious of things in your field of awareness, including sounds, sights, smells, and even the emotional signals being given off by others. But most important, a mindfulness pause enables a person to notice what is going on in their own mind and what physical sensations are being felt in various parts of their body.

Being mindful is to deliberately and purposefully pay attention to the present moment, and to fill the mind with one specific point of focus. The immediate benefits of doing so are numerous and integrated:

- Full concentration on the task or problem at hand (or of others with whom you are engaging).
- A sense of stillness and calm as anything other than the specific point of focus is channeled away.
- Increased cognitive processing power as more of the working memory is concentrated on the specific point of focus.
- Decreases in emotional outbursts, reactive actions, and regrettable words spoken.

- Higher quality decision making resulting from cognitive focus and fewer reactionary decisions or decisions made in fear or under stress.

- Reduced levels of stress and the associated health benefits that come with this, including lower blood pressure and decreased risks for heart disease, diabetes, obesity, and Alzheimer's disease.

There is an inherent self-regulatory aspect to mindfulness as one takes purposeful control over brain, body, thoughts, and emotions. This comes from the awareness and gathering of disparate and abundant bodily sensations, thoughts, and feelings that evolves into a body-mental-emotional integration and unification. When such an alignment is achieved, a sense of internal self-integrity surfaces.

As Frank J. Ninivaggi wrote in *Psychology Today* (April 2018), this sense of self-integrity "reflects a mind that is clear, openly receptive, balanced, poised, steady, and fluidly mobile without a fixed bottom line (e.g., the need to reach a fixed conclusion) at any moment."

Mindfulness is the self-regulation of:

- Attention
- Sensory awareness
- Perception
- The forming of emotions and thoughts
- Thinking
- Performance
- Actions

- Your decision-making process

The self-regulation of attention is a difficult challenge for most, but it is essential to the mindfulness process. This is the primary technique for accessing and managing thoughts, feelings, actions, performance, and your internal decision-making process.

As you see here, mindfulness is not just about taking a break and focusing on your breathing pattern. That is merely one technique. It is also about being fully present in the moment and leveraging the full power of your brain to deal with the challenges, people, problems, or tasks at hand.

Mindfulness has deep roots in the meditation practices of both Hinduism and Buddhism, as well as similar practices in Jewish, Islamic, and Orthodox Christian faiths. However, incorporating mindfulness practices into one's daily life requires no religious belief. Likewise, mindfulness is not counter to any personal religious beliefs or practices.

Some research has suggested that over 60% of a person's thoughts each day are negative or stress-inducing (and for some people this figure might be 80% to 90%). Over time, a daily mindfulness practice gradually reduces the number of rambling, discursive thoughts generated within the mind. If 60% (or more) of these wandering and sprawling thoughts are negative, then perhaps one of the utmost benefits of mindfulness is the reduction of such mentally and emotionally disturbing thoughts.

One other fundamental principle of mindfulness — in addition to focus and attention regulation, openness to the present and immediate experience, curiosity, and acceptance of the present moment — is the nonjudgmental awareness of one's own sensations, emotions, feelings, and thoughts. The key word here is nonjudgmental.

Self-judging of one's feelings, emotions, and thoughts tends to be highly and overly critical. (When was the last time you congratulated yourself for feeling good, joyous, or happy?) Such self-criticism leads to self-inflicted stress, thus hampering the ability to stay within a mindful mode. Being aware of your feelings, emotions, and thoughts without judging these as good or bad enables you to cognitively process these sensations and thoughts without instinctively acting upon them. This, in turn, leads to stress reduction, less fixedness in thought and emotional response, and an improved ability to become calm and relaxed, all of which enhances your decision-making capabilities.

What Sciences Says About Mindfulness

"Over the past ten or 12 years, there has been a vibrant interest in sectors of the neuroscience community in studying the impact of meditation, and now we have the tools," notes Richard Davidson, a psychologist at the University of Wisconsin Madison, in an article in *The Daily Beast*. Also the founder of the university's Center for Healthy Minds, Davidson said, "We can look at brain structure and function and study people repeatedly over time to see how prioritizing mindfulness and meditation impact the brain and change behavior and experience."

Davidson and other neuroscience researchers have begun to discover positive effects on the brain from mindfulness. In a meta-analysis study reported in *Brain and Cognition* in October 2016, researchers found that as few as eight weeks of mindfulness practice can produce long-term structural changes in brain architecture. According to the authors of the report, "Demonstrable functional and structural changes in the prefrontal cortex, cingulate cortex, insula, and hippocampus are similar to changes described in studies on traditional meditation practices."

The work of Jon Kabat-Zinn at the University of Massachusetts Medical School largely sparked today's modern thinking on mindfulness. He developed the school's Mindfulness-Based Stress Reduction (MBSR) programs to help patients deal with chronic pain. By getting patients to adopt a mindful approach to pain management, Kabat-Zinn found he could relieve their mental distress and help to improve overall functioning.

His documented successes led to mindfulness being incorporated into a wide range of cognitive and behavioral approaches by other researchers and medical practitioners. This resulted in mindfulness-based treatment approaches for depression, anxiety, addiction, post-traumatic stress disorder (PTSD), Obsessive-Compulsive Disorder (OCD), and even borderline personality disorder. Mindfulness centers and clinics now dot the landscape across the country and worldwide.

More recently, neuroscientists started investigating the links between mindfulness and brain architecture and brain function. This moved the thinking of mindfulness from a therapeutic practice used as a recovery technique for a range of emotional and mental issues to a tool and methodology for improving cognitive performance, reducing the impact of stressful events and situations, and regulating emotional reactions.

Scientific studies have shown measurable brain changes resulting from a mindfulness meditation commitment of around 20 minutes a day.

In one study from Canada, researchers proved that 25 minutes of mindfulness meditation generated greater improvement in brain function and energy levels than 25 minutes of quiet reading. The study also showed that mindfulness meditation specifically boosts the brain's executive function and cognitive abilities linked to goal-directed behavior. In addition, the study revealed that mindfulness meditators had a better ability to control knee-jerk emotional reactions, habitual thinking patterns, and actions

Today there are mindfulness educational and training programs for business leaders, employees, government officials, prisoners, athletes, medical professionals, combat soldiers, and countless other professions and groups.

Neuroimaging has shown that mindfulness practices modify neural circuits in the brain involved in the regulation of negative emotions. This is one of the many physical changes in the brain detected as a result of mindfulness and mindfulness meditation practices. Studies have also consistently shown that cognitive behavior therapy (CBT), one type of mindfulness practice used by therapists, changes dysfunctions of the nervous system.

As counterintuitive as it may seem, short breaks are highly productive in the workplace. One study showed that 20 minutes of yoga could significantly improve brain functioning. Another confirmed that quick naps boost memory. Another study showed that 52 minutes of intense work following by a 17-minute break is the ideal work pattern. All of the studies highlight the importance of recuperation time for the brain to achieve peak cognitive performance.

An additional good reason for taking short breaks and moving around a bit throughout the work day comes from another study at UCLA. Adding to previous research showing excessive sitting increases the risks for heart disease, diabetes, and shorter lifespans, this 2018 study used MRI scans to confirm that the medium temporal lobe, which creates new memories, was thinner in people who spent more time sitting. A short break that includes some physical movement will get more blood pumping to the brain, improving cognitive performance when you return to the next task or join the next meeting.

Additionally, for those of you who spend the preponderant portion of the day sitting at a desk or in meetings, the last thing you should do is flop down in front of the television when you get home. Better alternatives include a pit stop at the gym or a short stroll around the neighborhood or in a nearby park.

You may think that having a wandering, roaming mind is not normal. Don't worry; it is absolutely normal. We just do not tell one another about our wandering minds, so many feel that theirs is unusual. Unfortunately, wandering minds are not as happy as focused minds.

While research into the impact of wandering minds is still in its infancy, some studies are already showing causal linkages. A 2010 study reported in the journal *Science* showed that mind wandering leads to negative moods. A more recent study in 2017 revealed that seemingly innocent daydreams and fantasizing about the future could lead to depressive symptoms over time.

There are other significant drawbacks to a wandering mind: reading comprehension, memory recall, and cognitive control over emotions all decrease. Outside of creative activities like brainstorming, innovation, and artistic pursuits like writing and design, where daydreaming can be a powerful tool, focus is the best mental mode of operation for most tasks and decisions. It is definitely starting to be accepted by many in the neuroscientific community that learning to focus the mind has a lot of benefits.

The authors of a 2010 study reported in *Science* concluded that, "A human mind is a wandering mind and a wandering mind is an unhappy mind." Unfortunately, we all have wandering minds.

While there are many junk products, apps, videos, and books related to mindfulness on the market, these do not negate the verifiable benefits scientifically proven by respected and stalwart scientists and researchers. Even the National Institute of Health has chimed in, stating that some research suggests practicing mindfulness meditation can reduce blood pressure, symptoms of irritable bowel syndrome, anxiety, depression, insomnia, fibromyalgia, psoriasis, and post-traumatic stress disorder.

Becoming Mindful

Mindfulness is an exercise in focus. The point of the focus can be relaxation, emotional control, interpersonal interaction, cognitive problem solving, or decision making. Astute individuals use mindfulness in each of these situations, as well as many others.

The brain is wired to think. It is not possible to get the brain to stop thinking, much less to get it to stop thinking about something stressful. The only choice we have is to exert control over the brain through the deliberate practice of focusing attention on one specific thing at a time (mindfulness) to prevent it from being activated by other, stressful factors.

The tricky part is deciding to become mindful. We are so used to operating in autopilot mode, rushing from one activity or task to another, that we have no internal mechanism to remind us to pause and become fully present occasionally.

This is where technology can help. I have an app on my phone that sends me a simple notification message at random seven times a day. The message reads: *Am I mind full or mindful?* It is the one app that I allow to continue sending me notifications throughout the day. Although I do not receive these messages when I set my phone to airplane mode, usually at least one such reminder is waiting for me when I switch out of airplane mode. These messages create seven moments each day to remind me to pause, reflect on what I am doing and thinking, and recalibrate into a mindful state if necessary.

An ongoing mindfulness practice eventually leads to an enhanced ability to become aware of your own autopilot tendencies and thoughts. This provides you with the option of choosing a different way to respond or act, particularly if any of your habitual tendencies often lead to mistakes, regrets, or interpersonal relationship issues.

If you think that a mindful breathing practice has nothing to do with the workplace, consider the Navy SEALs. Facing some of the most stressful workplace conditions one can imagine, the SEALs use a four-part breathing sequence called Box Breathing. It is a technique that can be done in five minutes:

1) Find a comfortable chair or lie down.
2) Inhale for four seconds.
3) Hold the air in your lungs for four seconds.
4) Exhale for four seconds, emptying all the air in your lungs.
5) Hold your lungs empty for four seconds (no inhalation).
6) Repeat for five minutes, or as long as necessary to feel refocused and relaxed.

Personally, I find that taking three to four deep, purposeful breaths using the Box Breathing pattern during any stressful moments provides me with a sense of calm and the perspective I need to handle any situation more contemplatively and with full focus. Since I use a shortened version of this technique, I count between eight and ten at each step.

One of the most valuable benefits of becoming mindful, particularly during moments of high stress or difficult decision making, is that mindfulness opens the possibility of choices. An array of choices and options appear in mindful moments because opting to pause prevents habitual, knee-jerk responses from automatically surfacing and taking over. Removing yourself from autopilot mode helps prevent reactive decisions and responses. A mindfulness breather enables your conscious thoughts to hold sway over unconscious, instinctive, and automatic reactions.

Mindfulness also helps prevent over-reacting to non-emergency situations, such as the daily fire-fighting activities facing many people in the workplace. A mindful pause helps distinguish a minor brushfire from a three-alarm crisis. Equally as important, a moment of mindfulness helps prevent the kind of reactions that turn minor brushfires into unmitigated disasters threatening performance, results, and interpersonal relationships.

Mindfulness is a journey, not a destination. It is not something to be added to your daily to-do list, checked off when completed, and then forgotten about until the next day. It is something that is ideally integrated into your daily life and thus practiced (and experienced) throughout each and every day.

Mindfulness works best when inculcated into a person's standard operating procedures, something that becomes as automatic as tapping car brakes when a traffic light turns red. Mindfulness is a means of living a fully contented professional and personal life, with increased confidence in one's decisions, thoughts, and actions.

For those of us who are not Buddhist monks meditating in the hills above Dharamshala, cognitive control is the exception, not the rule. At least until we start to implement the tried and proven techniques of mindfulness skills (see chapters 8 and 9). But, like any skill, mindfulness proficiency can be learned, practiced, improved, and achieved.

Moving into mindfulness is just a matter of pausing when elevated stress has us emotionally worked up, taking a few deep breaths, and asking ourselves: *what are the best possible thoughts, emotions, actions, and decisions for this situation here in the present moment?*

Re-Energizing vs. Tuning Out

Thinking can be exhaustive. Cognitive contemplation is mentally draining. Problem solving, decision making, planning, being creative, negative thoughts, and even daydreaming are all mentally tiring activities.

When physical tiredness sets in, accidents and errors start to happen. When mental exhaustion surfaces, bad decisions are made, negative thoughts are voiced, and emotional outbursts spew with volcanic thunder.

When you are mentally tired, you likely do not have any energy to spare. And it takes energy to listen to one's spouse, deal with teenage angst or disruption, and even to focus on a televised sporting event.

So, how should you cope with life when mentally exhausted?

The only way to replenish physical energy is through rest and nutrition. The same holds true for mental energy. The best way to rest your brain is through mindfulness or meditation. Mindfulness exercises allow the brain to re-energize and the mind to refresh, refocus, and return to purposeful contemplation.

First, unwind (but don't vegetate). Go for a short walk, knock an easy task off your "honey-do" list, or even meditate. Whatever you do, take some time for yourself first and replenish your mental energy stores.

Now you are ready to engage with others. When doing so, continue to focus on your breathing to keep your thoughts from wandering. Pay full attention by listening reflectively. Play back some or all of what the other person is saying in your own words to keep you focused and grounded. Reply with relevant questions, seeking to understand more fully before responding.

The point of mental relaxation is not to get away from it all. The purpose is to prepare and refresh yourself mentally to enable you to return fully back into life. Mindfulness doesn't end at relaxation. It begins there. A bout of mental relaxation provides just enough stability to see what is happening in your mind and to gently inquire about its state.

This is why mindfulness is considered by many as a crucial practice for mental health. It gives you a chance to perform a quick health check on your mind. As such, it is just like when you slowly move your muscles to check for aches or when you pause to contemplate that queasiness in your stomach as part of your daily bodily health routine.

Mindful Focus

The workplace environment for most of us is one of constant distractions and interruptions. Hence, our natural inclination is to resort to a mode of multitasking. While this may be fine for simple tasks, such as deleting junk email while listening to a conference call, multitasking is the curse of focus and making good decisions.

Using a mindfulness mode increases focus, pushes away distractions, and enhances productivity and creativity. A mindfulness approach to increased focus entails:

1. Eliminating all potential distractions, including closing the email and Internet message programs on your computer and setting your mobile phone device to airplane mode. Close your door if you have one (and have a Do Not Disturb sign on it if culturally acceptable in your organization).

2. Ensuring you have sufficient water, coffee, tea, or other drinks to last at least an hour.

3. Using purposeful breathing to prepare your mind to concentrate.

4. Clearing out all thoughts and ruminations, including the mind's chatter about all the other tasks you could be doing (write these down for later reference if necessary to help clear your working memory space).

5. Taking two to five minutes to totally focus on the task at hand, remembering to include the most desirable outcome, or to picture what success will look like, i.e., "I will finish the first draft of this report before lunch."

6. Getting to work. If it is a task that will take several hours to complete, get up and take a short break every 75 minutes or so. Movement creates an increased circulation of blood, which is good for the brain. Use this time to replenish liquid supplies, grab a few minutes of fresh air, and think of something pleasurable.

However, do not access email or engage in conversations that are likely to mentally distract you from returning wholly focused on the task at hand. You do not want anything cluttering up your precious working memory space.

CHAPTER 6

The Impact of Mindfulness on Decision Making

Harried thinking can cause huge mistakes. When you feel out of control, or compelled to make decisions under immense time pressure, chances are the most optimal decisions will not be made.

Yes, business pressures and demands by others (customers, bosses, colleagues, etc.) often result in insufficient time to make an optimal decision. But how hard and firm are these deadline pressures? Most are arbitrarily set by someone, which also means they can be arbitrarily changed if a satisfactory reason is given.

It is not always possible to make wholly reasoned and highly analyzed decisions, especially given the pressures and busyness of the typical workplace. But it is always important to ask yourself and others: *can we make an optimal decision without slowing down and being entirely focused on the task or decision at hand?* More times than not, the answer is no.

There can be strategic advantages in "slowing down to speed up." Slowing down the decision-making process enables better decisions to be made. It also allows time for more significant input and participation in the decision-making process by all relevant team members and stakeholders. This, in turn, leads to greater buy-in for the eventual decision and doing so often means that actual implementation is speeded up and that fewer time-consuming course corrections are required. In the end, well thoughtout decisions lead to better and more fruitful actions and quicker implementation periods.

On the other hand, what if the deadline is firm and unchangeable? This is where mindfulness acceptance comes in and you strive to make the most optimal decision you can within the time constraints given. The questions you need to ask in these situations are:

> *How can we make the most optimal decision within the allotted time?*
>
> *How can we ensure the right people are entirely focused on this task or this decision for the duration of the decision-making process?*

Being mindful, meaning being fully present and aware of your own thoughts and feelings, helps you better know and understand when you are struggling to make decisions and the real causes behind these struggles. Recognizing your struggles and being aware of your thought patterns, feelings, and emotions are critical steps in making positive and meaningful personal change.

Another reason for mindfully moving into an optimistic state when making decisions is that optimism promotes the production of the neurotransmitter dopamine. This chemical not only makes us happy, it also promotes curiosity and a willingness to learn.

A study in Europe mapping the brains of people during puzzle-solving activities found that the moment of inspiration (the so-called aha! moment) when each puzzle was correctly solved was produced by an influx of dopamine into the nucleus accumbens region of the brain. This part of the brain, active throughout the process of problem solving, is part of the dopamine network that is triggered when we receive a reward.

Hence, there is now scientific proof that optimism, by increasing the production of dopamine, can lead to more rewarding puzzle solving and decision making.

Recent research by the INSEAD Business School revealed that increased mindfulness reduces the tendency to allow unrecoverable prior costs, known as sunk-cost bias, to influence current decisions. The study also found that just 15 minutes of mindfulness meditation can lead to more rational thinking when making business decisions.

Participants in the study used mindfulness meditation to reduce focus and thinking on the past and the future, to enable decisions based on information known in the current moment. This type of rational, present-moment thinking led to improved and expedited decision making. It resulted in better decisions and also prevented decisions from being over-analyzed for weeks.

Taking a mindful pause, whether this is a short meditation session or a clearing-the-head walk in nature, can lead to a more rewarding and effective decision-making process. Clearing the mind is an excellent remedy for the constant bombardment of information and data sent your way each and every day.

The key to truly developing the sharp focus that you need to make important or critical decisions requires thinking, analyzing, and evaluating on a deeper level. Cognitive improvement is only possible when we slow down, stop allowing technology and others to constantly interrupt us, and mindfully practice focusing on the task, information, or people with whom we are engaged.

These are the things that mindful decision makers do differently:

1. Do not multitask.

2. Cancel electronic notifications and set smartphones to airplane mode for extended periods of the day.

3. Use purposeful breathing as a stress reliever and to drive increased oxygen and blood to their brain.

4. Pause before responding.

5. Focus on the positives.

6. Constantly observe their thoughts and emotions nonjudgmentally.

7. Pay close attention to their breathing patterns.

8. Place importance on self-care, especially in terms of stress control and alleviation.

9. Practice being a good listener.

10. Use mindfulness techniques frequently and regularly throughout the work day.

There are many ways to attain more in-depth and more frequent moments of mindfulness. Reducing or stopping multitasking is one of the best places to start. In the next chapter, we will share some of the other proven benefits of mindfulness.

CHAPTER 7

Benefits of Mindfulness and Meditation

In many ways, mindfulness techniques, particularly mindful meditation practices, help create much-needed headspace. But that is not the only benefit of mindfulness, as this chapter will highlight.

According to a survey in the U.K. by the Mental Health Foundation, over 80% of the adult population agrees that the pace of modern life is a major cause of stress, unhappiness, and illness. There is little doubt that each of us could become healthier and more content if we could frequently switch off and slow down.

Being constantly stuck in overdrive is not living. Eventually, the body and brain will tire and break down. Neither are machines designed to operate at elevated levels day after day after day. Mindfulness helps us pause long enough to create some space in our lives — and in our minds — in order to preempt unhelpful thoughts and behavior patterns and to enable better (and different) choices and decisions.

Stanford Graduate School of Business lecturer Leah Weiss teaches a program called Leading with Mindfulness and Compassion. She believes mindfulness in the workplace is vital today as "nothing provides more opportunities than the workplace for us to feel discouraged, disappointed, bored, overwhelmed, envious, embarrassed, anxious, irritated, outraged, and afraid to say what really feel."

In her book, *How We Work: Live Your Purpose, Reclaim Your Sanity, and Embrace the Daily Grind*, she describes three kinds of mindfulness:

> Embodiment — having mindfulness of the body. Being aware of your body as you go through the day, as the body is a principal source of information on pain and the physical manifestations of emotions.
>
> Metacognition — the ability to know what we are experiencing as we experience it. It is the ability to observe one's own thoughts, actions, and emotions in the moment. In her words, "By separating the data — what is really happening vs. our interpretation of what is happening — we can find places where we are spinning stories that are not helpful to us, others, or our productivity."
>
> Focus — the ability to direct our attention where we want it. Improving the ability to focus requires retraining the mind to notice in the moment when we are distracted and return to the object of focus.

Mindfulness Impact on Stress and Emotions

Mindfulness is proving to be a key weapon against stress.

A study published in the journal *Psychiatry Research* reported that anxious people who took a mindfulness course where they learned several different strategies reacted to stress better and had a lower hormonal and inflammatory response to stress than people who did not practice mindfulness.

The folks in the study who learned meditative practices, such as breath awareness, body scan meditations, and gentle yoga, responded feeling less stress than the study's control group. More important, from a scientific viewpoint, these people also had blood measurements of ACTH, a stress hormone released in the brain and then into the bloodstream, lower than that measured in the control group. Additionally, their blood markers of inflammation, called pre-inflammatory cytokines, were lower as well.

"We have objective measures in the blood that they did better in a provoked situation," stated lead research author Dr. Elizabeth Hoge, associate professor of psychology at Georgetown University Medical Center. "It is really strong evidence that mindfulness meditation not only makes them feel better, but helps them be more resilient to stress."

Meditation has also been shown to reduce stress hormones, such as cortisol, while increasing endorphins, dopamine, and other hormones that lower stress and slow the aging process. Meditation also lessens inflammation, which damages and ages cells.

Mindfulness is extremely useful in helping us deal with difficult emotions and situations or events that tend to trigger strongly felt negative emotions. Mindfulness is used to find the gap between a triggering event or comment and our usual conditioned response. This enables us to use this pause to collect ourselves and change our customary responses accordingly. In other words, mindfulness helps us learn to make better choices and to reduce habitual reactions that escalate situations or lead to regret.

By taking a mindful moment, we get to nonjudgmentally acknowledge what we are feeling and to spot our habitual reactions before they get put into motion. Then we can decide on a different and healthier course of action than usual.

Additionally, research by neuroscientist Richard Davidson showed that people who meditate regularly have an enhanced ability to respond empathetically to others without feeling overwhelmed.

Mindfulness Impact on Overall Health

The practice of mindfulness has been scientifically linked to a number of positive benefits, including lowering stress, reducing chronic pain, and boosting overall health and wellbeing. There is also significant research showing that mindfulness can help regulate appetite in a healthy way, reduce alcohol consumption, and help those who wish to quit smoking.

After reviewing dozens of studies analyzing eight different types of meditation and their effects on various heart disease risk factors, the American Heart Association says meditation may help against heart disease. To be clear, the AHA says that meditation can be considered *in addition* to existing standard treatment for heart problems, which include lowering cholesterol, losing weight, and cessation of smoking.

"Our clear message is that meditation may be a reasonable (additional) intervention, but we specifically do not want people to rely on meditation or other such adjunctive interventions in place of proven therapies," notes Dr. Glenn Levine, chair of the AHA and American College of Cardiology task force on clinical practice guidelines.

The studies analyzed showed that meditation might help to lower some of the risk factors for heart diseases, such as reducing stress and hypertension. As noted above, lowering stress can reduce the levels of stress hormones in the body, which have been linked to a higher rate of heart attacks. Also, keeping blood pressure low can dampen the risk of heart trouble.

One of the research studies analyzed by the American Heart Association was undoubtedly a study released in 2009 that had followed 200 patients for an average of five years. In that study, researchers concluded that high-risk patients who meditated cut their risk of heart attacks, strokes, and deaths from all causes roughly in half compared with a group of similar patients given more conventional education about healthy diet and lifestyle.

The meditators in this study also tended to remain disease-free longer. Also, they reduced their systolic blood pressure reading (the upper number, which measures the pressure in blood vessels when the heart beats) by five points on average. An earlier study of high-risk patients, many of them overweight or obese, also found that meditation, along with conventional medications, could help reduce blood pressure.

Chronic inflammation is the long-term, runaway activation of the immune system, even in the absence of injury or infection. Such inflammation is at the core of a wide range of health problems, including heart disease, diabetes, cancer, stroke, depression, and Alzheimer's disease. Mindfulness reduces inflammation by impacting changes in the brain's functional connectivity, according to researchers at Carnegie Mellon University.

Brain scans of participants in this study revealed that meditation increased functional connectivity between two brain areas that typically work in opposition — the default mode network, which is involved in mind wandering and internal reflection, and the executive attention network, which is key to planning, attention, and decision making. Additionally, blood samples of the participants who had gone through a three-day mindfulness training program had lower levels of Interleukin-6, a biomarker of inflammation.

The researchers concluded that the changes seen in functional brain connectivity, resulting from the mindfulness training program, appeared to help the brain better manage stress, a known inflammation trigger. Hence, the reduction in stress hormones was directly responsible for the reduced levels of inflammation.

A Brown University study published in the *American Journal of Health Behavior* found a link between a high level of mindfulness and healthy levels of glucose. An unhealthy amount of glucose in the blood is one risk factor for developing diseases like Type 2 diabetes and other aspects of metabolic syndrome. These results are in line with other studies that have shown that mindfulness lowers the risk of obesity and helps people feel a greater sense of self-control over their lives.

In another study at Brown University, people who were not mindful were 34% more likely to be obese. They were also more likely to have increased abdominal fat. Additionally, even those who were not obese as children, but who had become obese as adults, had lower mindfulness scores than people who were not obese in either childhood or adulthood.

Since mindfulness is a skill that can be learned and practiced, those at risk for diabetes and obesity due to lifestyle choices or genetic disposition have a skill set available to them to decrease their odds of illness and major health issues should they want. Mindfulness may, in fact, be the best methodology for changing habits that result in a better life.

Lastly, here is more good news about mindfulness meditation. A 2017 study that analyzed immune system cells discovered that people who regularly meditated had slower epigenetic clocks, a DNA marker of aging. This study used a very small sample size and the results need to be replicated and confirmed in a more extensive study. But it was the first time that a connection between regular mindfulness meditation and a slowing of the aging process had been seen.

However, what is known through other studies is that cumulative chronic stress speeds up the epigenetic clock. Hence, since mindfulness meditation is a proven stress reducer, the logical hypothesis would be that regular mindfulness meditation is likely to make the epigenetic clock tick at a slower pace.

Mindfulness Impact on Brain Health

Closely related to everyone's apprehensions about the natural aging process we face as sentient beings are perhaps even more substantial concerns and fears related to cognitive decline and associated issues such as dementia and Alzheimer's disease.

As Sandra Bond Chapman, the founder and director of the Center for BrainHealth at the University of Texas at Dallas, told the Chicago Tribune in early 2018, "Alzheimer's now tops heart disease and cancer when it comes to our fear factor about diseases."

Researchers from the University of British Columbia reviewed data from more than 20 studies on how mindfulness impacts the brain and brain health. While they determined that significant changes occur in eight different parts of the brain as a result of practicing mindfulness, two of these regions are of momentous importance:

1) The anterior cingulate cortex (ACC), which is responsible for self-control and focus. It also influences the ability to resist distractions and avoid impulsive actions. Additionally, the ACC is in control of flexibility, and people who have problems in this brain area are known to

stick to ineffective problem-solving strategies instead of adapting and adjusting their approaches.

2) The hippocampus, which is in charge of resilience in the face of setbacks and challenges. Unfortunately, the hippocampus is readily damaged by stress and thus benefits from stress-reducing activities.

Researchers from the University of California Davis Center for Mind and Brain spent seven years following a group of people who regularly meditated. The authors of the study report concluded that meditation can enhance mental abilities and protect against age-related cognitive decline. It is the first study to provide evidence that continued meditation practice over an extended period of time is associated with long-lasting improvements in sustained attention.

The ability to focus, of course, is a trait that often begins to falter with age. A decline in focus ability and attention span is usually a precursor to other adverse cognitive effects of aging.

As the researchers wrote in their paper (study results were published in the *Journal of Cognitive Enhancement* in April 2018), "The present study suggests that intensive and continued meditation is associated with enduring improvements in sustained attention, supporting the notion that the cognitive benefits of dedicated mental training may persist over the long term when promoted by a regimen of continued practice."

According to a meta-analysis of all the existing studies on the subject, a simple mindfulness meditation routine can have profound, physical effects on the brain in only eight weeks.

The study, published in the scientific journal *Brain and Cognition* in October 2016, examined 30 studies that used MRI brain scans to measure the physical changes in the brain resulting from meditation practices. Here is the summary of the study results:

> Associated brain changes, in terms of activity levels and volume and connectivity changes, have been reported in the prefrontal cortex (a region associated with conscious decision making, emotional regulation, and other functions), the insula (which represents internal body states among other things), the cingulate cortex (decision making), the hippocampus (memory), and the amygdala (emotion).

These results strongly indicate that a mere eight weeks of daily mindfulness meditation is sufficient to rewire the brain to enhance greater focus, increased emotional control, and promote higher quality, more thoughtful decision making.

A group of researchers at UCLA have also been studying the effects of meditation on brain aging. One study they conducted examined how longtime meditators at age 50 compared on cognitive tests with 50-year olds who do not meditate. They discovered a vast difference: those who had regularly meditated for years had brains that were estimated to be around 7.5 years younger than their contemporaries who did not meditate.

The researchers conducting this study concluded that, "These findings seem to suggest that meditation is beneficial for brain preservation, effectively protecting against age-related atrophy with a consistently slower rate of brain aging throughout life."

It does not take much time meditating to generate measurable results. "We've shown in the laboratory that meditating for a half-hour a day for two weeks is enough to produce changes in the brain," says Richard Davidson, a psychologist at the University of Wisconsin Madison. "Most people recognize that if you go to the gym for two weeks and work out every day with a personal trainer you'll feel a difference. But those changes aren't going to persist unless you keep exercising. Meditation is very similar. It's a form of mental exercise. And once you begin to experience beneficial changes, it will inspire you to continue practicing for the rest of your life."

"In most parts of the world today, people practice some kind of personal physical hygiene," says Davidson. "My aspiration is that people will care for their minds in the same way. They will engage in simple practices that will be disseminated very widely. I am convinced the world would be a very different place if we can cross that tipping point."

Impact on Brain Function

According to science, here are five things that happen to the brain during meditation:

1. Cortisol (a stress hormone) levels are lowered.
2. Brainwave activity increases.
3. Dopamine, the so-called feel-good neurotransmitter, is released into the brain and body, resulting in a state of deep relaxation.
4. Grey matter in the hippocampus (the region of the brain crucial for learning and memory) increases.
5. Re-wiring within the brain occurs, creating new neural connections.

Scientific research has also revealed that meditation increases the cortical thickness in the hippocampus, the part of the brain that runs memory and influences the ability to learn new things. It is also the region of the brain where Alzheimer's disease wrecks so much havoc. So anything that helps strengthen this region of the brain might be beneficial in warding off the onset of Alzheimer's.

Mindfulness has also been shown to help with long-term memory. Researchers have recently discovered a strong connection between memory recall and the conditions under which the memory was initially formed. The study, reported in *Scientific Reports* (May 2018), revealed that calm surroundings contribute to greater memory retention, and that moments of silence actually help to galvanize and strengthen memories. This allows them to be recalled with greater detail, even over time.

Hence, the moments immediately following an event or the intake of new information can impact the quality of the memory that is formed. Thus, having a quiet moment of mindfulness after receiving significant information is likely to do wonders for how well you recall the details of this information later. It is another reason to schedule a few minutes of mindfulness in between your back-to-back meetings.

The amygdala, the section of the brain where fear resides, has less grey matter in meditators compared to those who do not meditate. When the grey matter reduces in the amygdala, it correspondingly thickens in the prefrontal cortex area, where awareness and decision making are centered. Long-term meditators are found to be less fearful than non-meditators. They are also seen to have slower reaction times to emotional situations as their larger prefrontal cortexes take the time to respond less reactively.

A study released in May 2017 showed that three months of mindfulness meditation practice leads to a noticeable shift in how the brain allocates attention. The ability to release thoughts that magically pop into the mind is a skill learned through mindful meditation. Apparently, that skill frees the brain to better process rapidly changing things, such as emotional facial expressions and situational events.

According to study results at the University of California Davis, gains developed through intensive meditation training in the ability to sustain attention are maintained up to seven years later.

Practicing yoga or mindfulness for just 25 minutes a day can boost the brain's executive functions, according to a study released by the University of Waterloo in Canada. Doing either on a daily basis also improved cognitive abilities linked to goal-directed behavior and the ability to control knee-jerk emotional responses, routine thinking patterns, and habitual actions.

Accumulating evidence from a wide range of studies shows that yoga is good for the brain, as well as the body and overall health of yoga practitioners. Yoga has been used in the treatment of anxiety conditions, depression, insomnia, eating disorders, and other health-related issues. Like mindfulness, yoga helps to reduce chronic stress, which is connected to many physical and mental ailments. Yoga is also known to help reduce the stress hormone cortisol, thus helping to improve mood and emotional regulation.

In addition to helping to keep the body young and in better shape, yoga does wonders for the brain as well. In a 2017 study published in the journal *International Psychogeriatrics*, older adults (defined as 55+) with mild cognitive impairment spent 12 weeks either practicing Kundalini yoga or memory training. As expected, both groups showed memory improvements. However, the yoga group saw a boost in executive functioning and emotional resilience, which the researchers believed was possibly due to the chanting in this yoga method that strengthens visual and verbal skills.

Regular mindfulness meditation appears to make it easier to focus. "Hatha yoga and mindfulness meditation both focus the brain's conscious processing power on a limited number of targets like breathing and posing, and also reduce processing of nonessential information," notes Peter Hall, associate professor at the University of Waterloo. "These two functions might have some positive carryover effect in the near-term following the session, such that people are able to focus more easily on what they choose to attend to in everyday life."

Everyone has more cognitive stress today than ever before, and this often prevents or blunts the ability to focus on a given task, problem, situation, or decision. Several studies, such as the one from the University of Waterloo, are finding that mental training through mindfulness techniques can reinforce — and even rewire — the neural connections used to drive individual performance and decision making. By taking just ten minutes or so to mentally and mindfully prepare for the next task, while simultaneously giving the brain time to refresh and re-energize, we enhance our abilities to perform at peak levels effectively and efficiently.

In another byproduct finding from the University of Waterloo study, both mindfulness meditation and yoga were effective in improving individual energy levels.

Other Benefits

Incorporating mindfulness into one's life also usually results in greater awareness and appreciation of the beauty in life. Reducing busyness creates countless opportunities to notice and appreciate the chattering of birds, the colors of trees and flowers, a gentle breeze, and the smells of food cooking.

Raising our mindfulness levels also puts us more in tune with the feelings of others, helps us to notice and share in the joy a child or friend is feeling, and makes us more sensitive to the daily plights others are experiencing.

Getting outdoors and into nature (not the office parking lot!) is profoundly good for us. The proven effects of spending some time with nature include reducing stress, boosting happiness, and aiding creativity. Add one more item to the long list of positive health and wellbeing benefits that can be derived from basking in the glories of nature — attention span.

According to recent research, spending time in a nearby park or any other natural setting may double your focus and attention span. Even being able to view nature through windows for 40-60 seconds is enough to refresh the brain and increase attention capabilities.

And that's the beauty of mindfulness. You can be mindful anywhere and at any time you choose.

Now that you have a good grasp on the benefits of mindfulness and meditation, the next chapter will provide you tips on how you can readily shift into mindfulness, even at work.

CHAPTER 8

Shifting Into Mindfulness

There are many ways to shift from busyness and craziness into mindfulness. Each merely takes awareness that you are not fully present in the moment, followed by conscious and purposeful action to pause and become as close to fully present as possible.

The most basic mindfulness method is simply to pause, clear your mind of all but one single thought, and concentrate on your breathing. This can be done with eyes opened or closed, and I find either way works equally well.

The process is straightforward. Shift your attention to a predetermined thought or find something visual or auditory as a point of focus. At home, I will close my eyes, shift into a deeper breathing pattern, and listen acutely for the chirps and song notes of birds. In an airport standing or sitting around waiting to board a plane (something I do very frequently), I will keep my eyes open, again go into a deep breathing pattern, and focus on observing a worker on the tarmac.

You can even use smell and feelings as points of focus. Take a steaming cup of coffee or tea and hold this tightly in your hands. Segue into a deep breathing pattern and focus on the aroma emanating from your beverage. With each deep breath, feel the intensity of the warm cup on your hands and fingers or the powerful aroma filling your nostrils. After a minute or two of this, reward the peace and mindful presence you feel with a nice long sip of your brew.

Breathing and Go-To Words

If you want to focus solely on your breathing, an excellent technique is the box breathing technique used by U.S. Navy SEALs to stay calm and aware. Since your workplace or personal stress is unlikely to match that of a SEAL, chances are this breathing pattern technique will work for you as well.

I described this technique earlier (see page 99) and how I use it, so here is a shortened description of this breathing pattern. In box breathing, you count in four-second intervals as follows:

- Inhale for four seconds.
- Hold your breath for four seconds.
- Exhale for four seconds.
- Hold for four seconds.

Repeat this pattern for eight complete cycles, and in just over two minutes you should feel more energized, less stressed, and have greater clarity on whatever is going on around you or within you. Remember, you must focus only on your breathing during box breathing. If a thought enters your mind, simply let it flow in and then out like a receding ocean tide.

Box breathing balances the autonomic nervous system, which regulates involuntary body functions like temperature. It can also lower blood pressure, provide an almost immediate sense of calm, and increase alertness, energy, and motivation.

Personally, I often extend the box breathing technique to last between five and eight minutes, partially by increasing the interval counts from four to eight seconds. Doing this in my seat while others are still boarding a flight is a great way to remain calm and not get incensed by fellow passengers who violate the carry-on policies.

Another way to quickly shift into mindfulness is to have three or four "go-to" words that can bring forth potent visual images in your mind. Each word should represent an image that will help you counter or slow the rise of negative emotions. For me, when I start to feel myself getting angry, my go-to word is sunshine. It is hard (for me anyway) to continue getting angry when I have a picture of bright sunshine and clear blue skies in my mind.

Likewise, I use the word beach to conjure up a peaceful beach scene in the late afternoon when I need to bring forth peace and calmness into a moment that is starting to go elsewhere. If the image is strong enough, I can actually feel the cool ocean breeze blowing across my face and body.

Finally, when I am stuck creatively, usually due to distracting thoughts or unwanted interruptions, I use the word waterfall to fill my mind with an image of rushing and bubbling water cascading off a mountainside cliff and into a river below. After a few moments (usually 75 to 90 seconds) visualizing this scene, I am ready to be fully present in the real moment. Somehow this image of integrated power and unstoppable movement of water restarts my creative juices and propels me back into full creative concentration (and mindfulness) mode.

Naturally, these three words (sunshine, beach, and waterfall) may not have much relevance to you. Find your own words that can automatically surface meaningful images that will snap you into a mindfulness moment.

For those whose overly active brains have them struggling to get to sleep, transitioning into 5-15 minutes of mindfulness meditation is often the ticket to a good night's rest. Turn off the television and any music with lyrics and simply close your eyes while sitting or reclining horizontally.

Once you are comfortable, become perfectly still. Focus only on your breathing (inhaling through the nose and exhaling via the mouth) using the box breathing technique described above. If instrumental music helps soothe and calm you, feel free to have this playing softly in the background. Now head off to sleep.

Purposeful Rhythmic Breathing

We all breathe. Some 23,000 times or more a day. Automatically. Without thinking or consideration. And unless breathing becomes difficult due to a cold, injury, allergy, or a respiratory disease, most of us do not give breathing much thought.

So let's give it a thought. Many thoughts, in fact. Concentrated breathing, or what I call purposeful breathing, is also sometimes referred to as breathwork. Why? Because it takes concentration and work to focus solely on something you habitually do unconsciously and automatically.

"Breathing is life," notes Tim Altman, a respiratory therapist, naturopath, and sports coach in Australia. "It is the body function we perform more than any other, apart from the heartbeat."

Adds Altman, who works on breath coaching with groups and in the corporate sector, "Pretty much all of us breathe incorrectly, in that we over-breathe — both too often and with too much volume. This upsets the delicate balance in our respiratory system and reduces energy production. The implications of this are felt in all parts of our body.

In addition, breathing is the only automatic body function we have that we can consciously control with ease, and the same nervous system that controls our automatic functions also controls our response to stress. Therefore, by learning to breathe correctly, we can dramatically and positively influence all of the other automatic functions in the body, as well as our energy, mood, and stress levels."

Breathing more deeply and at a slower pace has numerous benefits, including relaxing tension in the body, calming nervous shaking, and decreasing blood pressure. Purposeful breathing helps you feel connected to your body, while simultaneously washing away the worries in your head and quieting the mind.

According to a recent study at Northwestern University, the way we breathe affects the way we think and feel. Researchers there discovered that the rhythm of breathing creates electrical activity in the brain, with the effect being slightly different depending on whether a person is inhaling or exhaling.

"One of the major findings of this study is that there is a dramatic difference in brain activity in the amygdala and hippocampus during inhalation compared with exhalation," reports Christina Zelano, assistant professor of neurology at Northwestern University Feinberg School of Medicine. "When you breathe in, we discovered you are stimulating the neurons in the olfactory cortex, amygdala, and hippocampus, all across the limbic system. When you inhale, you are, in a sense, synchronizing brain oscillations across the limbic network."

This is why breathing deeply calms the brain. It has to do with a cluster of neurons in the brainstem called the pacemaker for breathing. These neurons affect breathing, emotional states, and alertness. Scientists have found that this neural circuit causes us to be anxious when we breathe rapidly and calm when we breathe slowly. Hence, by changing our patterns of breathing, we can change our emotional states, as well as how we think and interact with the world.

When we do not breathe well, we do not feel well, either physically or mentally. Perhaps knowing this is what led the

American Institute of Stress to proclaim, "Abdominal breathing for 20 to 30 minutes each day will reduce anxiety and reduce stress."

Whether you call it abdominal breathing, diaphragmatic breathing, purposeful breathing, or simply deep breathing, a conscious breathing pattern of deep breaths increases the supply of oxygen to the brain. It also stimulates the parasympathetic nervous system, which promotes a state of calmness.

Breathing deeply means breathing less with your chest and more with your diaphragm. This is easy to determine. Place your right hand over your chest and your left hand over your navel. Take a normal breath. If only your right hand is moving, your breathing may be shallow. This can increase fatigue and anxiety. If your left hand is also moving, you are breathing deeply and properly.

There are lots of instructions on using the "right" posture to aid breathwork. This mostly applies to meditative sessions, not short bursts of purposeful breathing for moving into mindfulness. Personally, I am a big believer in comfort over structure, especially if I am going to be meditating for more than three to five minutes (my daily meditation sessions are 34 minutes).

Purposeful breathing, which can be done in conjunction with mindfulness meditation or on its own, has a profoundly rhythmic pattern to it. The key feature is to inhale and exhale greater than usual, with moments of pause between each inhalation and exhalation.

The process of purposeful breathing begins with a deep, slow inhalation that fills your lungs to capacity. Breathing in through the nostrils is best as this filters the air and is better for oxygen intake. Fill your belly and chest with air as your body starts to expand like an inflatable pool toy. Allow your shoulders and your abdomen to rise and fall with each respiratory cycle. By forcing your abdomen to expand, you will also be extending the diaphragm and pushing your ribs out.

As you exhale, push out all the air that you can, from both your lungs and your abdomen region. Use a little light force to exhale more deeply than usual. The exhale should be slightly longer than the inhale, as this slows the heart rate. Now pause and notice how your body feels emptied of oxygen. Remain still for a count of four to eight, then repeat the process beginning with another deep inhalation.

Throughout this process, focus as much as you can only on your breathing. Without a doubt, other thoughts will creep in, including "this is so boring." Simply cast aside these thoughts and refocus on your breathing. If your mind continues to wander, refocus by silently counting each step in the process: inhale (one, two, three, four, five, six), hold (one, two, three, four, five, six), exhale (one, two, three, four, five, six), and hold (one, two, three, four, five, six). As mentioned previously, the brain cannot process more than one thought at a time. When you are entirely focused on counting through each step in the purposeful breathing cycle, your brain cannot interrupt with its own thoughts or agenda.

One interesting point about inhalation through the nostrils. Breathing in slowly through the nose causes nerve fibers in the nasal passages to fire in a slow rhythm, prompting parts of the brain to do so as well. This is why people using slow nasal breathing enter a deeper meditative state than when they breathe at the same rate through their mouths.

One thing I like to do when practicing purposeful breathing during the workday is to go outside (or open a window if stuck inside) and listen for the sounds of birds chirping and singing. Of course, this does not work when I am visiting major metropolitan cities like New York (unless I can get to Central Park) or Tokyo (unless I find my way to the city's famed Shinjuku Gyoen Park).

Purposefully listening for bird sounds can even drown out road noise when I am wholly focused. Remember, the brain can only focus on one thing, so in effect it does not hear, or process, the traffic noise even though this is louder than the chirping and tweeting of the birds. I know the birds do not start singing just because I have stopped to listen. They are chirping away nonstop, whether I pause to hear them or not. Which just goes to prove, what you focus on listening for is what you will hear, if you are mindfully present.

Like any skill, purposeful breathing takes practice and repetition. Do not expect to master this in a week, no matter how simple it sounds. The brain does not appreciate being consciously controlled and it will fight back at first. Eventually, the brain comes to accept and appreciate the calmness and reduced stress that purposeful breathing brings, and eventually consents to this as the new normal.

Use the purposeful breathing technique whenever you need to switch into mindfulness and become more present with yourself, the people around you, and any circumstances or events.

Purposeful Breathing Exercises

"Using your breath to calm the body and mind is one of the most effective and powerful tools we as humans embody," notes Stuart Sandeman, a leading breath expert in the U.K. and founder of BreathPod.

He adds, "Your breath is a direct link to your autonomic nervous system. Your autonomic nervous system has two response states: sympathetic (your stress response often referred to as fight or flight response) and parasympathetic (your rest response, where you digest and repair)."

Naturally, when you are feeling overwhelmed, or in a state of stress, anxiety, confusion, or pressure, the sympathetic response state dominates your brain functions. Any of the purposeful breathing techniques below can help control your breathing pattern, slow down your heart rate, relax your muscles, re-balance, calm your mind, and quiet the parts of the autonomic nervous system generating the sympathetic response.

Dr. Andrew Weil developed the 4-7-8 breathing technique. It is a breathing pattern based on an ancient yoga technique call *pranayama*. Some practitioners believe this technique helps them fall asleep in a shorter amount of time. Others claim it can soothe a racing heart or calm frazzled nerves.

Prepare for this practice of controlled breathing by resting the tip of the tongue against the roof of the mouth. The tongue needs to remain in place throughout the breathing exercise, which takes some practice as it tends to move down during exhalation. Exhaling during 4-7-8 breathing can be more comfortable for some people when they purse their lips.

Here are the steps for 4-7-8 breathing, completing them counts as one cycle:

1. All the lips to part. Make a whooshing sound, exhaling completely through the mouth.
2. Close the lips and inhale silently through the nose while counting to four.
3. Hold your breath for a count of seven.
4. Make another whooshing exhale through the mouth for a count of eight, remembering to keep the tip of the tongue pressed lightly against the roof of the mouth.

Repeat his pattern four more times. The breath-holding period of seven seconds (or seven counts) is said to be most critical for this breathing exercise.

Another breathing exercise is alternate nostril breathing, called *Nadi Shodhana*. It is a powerful breathing technique that can help relax the mind, calm the nervous system, and clear nasal circulation. Here's how to do alternative nostril breathing:

1. Sit comfortably with the spine straight.
2. Close your eyes and take a few deep inhalations through both nostrils. Exhale through the nostrils.
3. Take the right hand and place the index and middle fingers between the eyebrows as a light anchor.
4. Gently close the right nostril with the right thumb and inhale slowly and deeply only through the left nostril for a count of five.
5. Hold your breath for a count of four or five.
6. Release the right nostril and close the left nostril with the right-hand ring finger.
7. Exhale slowly through the right nostril for a count of five.
8. Keeping the left nostril closed, inhale slowly and deeply through the right nostril for a count of five.
9. Pause after inhalation for a count of four or five. Release the left nostril and close the right nostril with the right thumb.

10. Exhale slowly through the left nostril for a count of five.

11. Inhale slowly and deeply through the left nostril for a count of five.

Repeat this alternate nostril breathing exercise five to ten times, breathing as slowly and deeply as possible. The process may be a bit awkward at first, but you should catch on quickly.

Our minds tend to wander during purposeful breathing exercises. This is particularly true for new practitioners of these techniques. One way to force the mind to concentrate on your breathing process is called square breathing. In this exercise, you draw an imaginary square in the air as you work through a purposeful breathing routine, as follows:

1. While inhaling slowly, count to four and draw the upward line of an imaginary square in the air.

2. Keeping your focus on the imaginary square, hold the inhalation for a count of four and draw the top line of the square in the air.

3. Exhale slowly to a count of four while drawing the downward line of the imaginary square in the air.

4. Hold your empty breath for a count of four while drawing the bottom line to complete he imaginary square.

Repeat this process up to 10-12 times, either with your eyes opened or closed. Picturing the imaginary square in the air as it is drawn helps prevent the mind from grasping onto other thoughts.

Another relaxation breathing technique is called Squish and Relax. The squish and relax exercise brings awareness to the body while relaxing tense muscles. For this breathing exercise, lie down with your eyes closed. As you inhale squish and squeeze every muscle in your body as tightly and firmly as you can.

Squish your toes and feet, tighten all the muscles in your legs, suck in your abdomen, squeeze your hands into fists, and raise your shoulders to your head. Hold yourself (and your breath) in this squished up position for a few seconds. Then, while exhaling, fully release your body and relax. Repeat this process three to four more times.

One very simple breathing exercise to help you move into a parasympathetic state is called the Double Calm Breath. The key here is to merely double the length of the exhale to the length of the inhale. For example:

1. Inhale for a count of four through your nose.
2. Exhale through pursed lips for a count of eight.
3. Inhale through the nose for a count of five.
4. Exhale through pursed lips for a count of ten.
5. Inhale for a count of six through the nose.
6. Exhale for a count of twelve.

In the Flow

In 1975, psychologist Mihály Csikszentmihályi first described what he called "flow" and what many of us think as "being in the zone." In this mental state, we are fully concentrated on a task at hand, and hours can fly by like minutes. Some describe this as a "rush" feeling, where all mental (and sometimes physical) energy is dispensed with singular purpose and focus.

Flow is a heightened state of mindfulness and feels exceedingly good when it happens. When flow occurs, it is the result of a perfect match between activity in the brain regions involved in attention and reward. When two brain networks synchronize their activity, it smooths the function of thinking, which explains why flow seems so effortless when you are experiencing it. In fact, thinking becomes so automatic and unconscious that you are not even aware of it.

Many athletes describe being "in the zone" as something that happens automatically without their thinking. That is absolutely true, as their conscious thinking is replaced by powerful unconscious thinking in a mindfulness state. Like athletes, anyone experiencing flow is "locked-in" and fully present.

Getting "into the zone" or "into flow" is one of the best outcomes of entering a mindfulness state, at least for me. This is why mindfulness is not an attempt at "getting away from it all," but rather a methodology for "getting fully into it all."

As Mihály Csikszentmihályi noted, "The best moments in our lives are not the passive, receptive, relaxing times. The best moments usually occur if a person's body or mind is stretched to its limits in a voluntary effort to accomplish something difficult and worthwhile."

Unfortunately, flow is hard to achieve and difficult to maintain for any length of time. However, the higher your mindfulness levels, the greater are the chances of slipping into flow.

Regular breaks during the workday also create opportunities to slip into mindfulness and flow. Here's advice from the *Harvard Business Review* (May 2018):

> Schedule 15-minute breaks at least once or twice a day to sit quietly in your office or take a walk. Commit to these breaks as you would any other meeting or appointment; if you don't schedule moments of quiet, something else will fill the time. Solitude gives you the space to reflect on where

your time is being spent. Try to get clarity on which meetings you should stop attending, which committees you should step down from, and which invitations you should politely decline.

As one who takes 10-15 minute "moments of silence" breaks regularly, I can tell you that these are quite happily very addictive. And very productivity enhancing as well.

Moving Into Mindfulness

Here are a dozen ways to move into mindfulness when you are feeling anxious, angry, stressed, or even just overwhelmed:

1. Admit to yourself exactly how you are feeling. Own these feelings nonjudgmentally.

2. Change your thinking from a "worst-case scenario" to an array of other possibilities and potential outcomes.

3. Take a walk, or engage in some other physical activity, to release the anxiety, anger, or other emotions before you act upon these.

4. Use one of your "go-to" words to conjure up a visualization that changes your thinking. If you do not have these words and images predetermined, then simply close your eyes and visualize yourself in a calm state.

5. Once your emotions and habitual reactions are in control (through mindful meditation or any of the four preceding actions), think through the situation with a greater focus on rationality. Focus on questions such as, *"Will this matter to me a week from now?"* and *"Am I willing to*

allow this person, these comments, or this situation ruin my internal peace?"

6. Listen to some soothing music or play a relaxing YouTube video.

7. Go get some fresh air. Being indoors can increase anxiety and anger due to a feeling of confinement. Go outside, even if for only a few minutes. Fresh air will likely help in calming you down, and the change of scenery often interrupts stressed, anxious, or angry thought processes.

8. Change the focus of your vision. Leave the situation. Look away from the other person. Walk out of the room. Go outside. Grab a coffee or a bite to eat. Just stop staring at the situation or person causing you to be upset.

9. Find a way to relax your body. The body tenses under stress and anger. Sit down and slowly stretch calf, leg, and shoulder muscles. If possible, lie down and slowly relax every part of your body. Start with the toes and work your way up to your jaw and facial muscles.

10. Write down what is troubling you. Write down how you are feeling and how you would like to react if there were no repercussions in doing so. Writing down negative thoughts and feelings helps to get them out of your head. And sometimes, crumbling up the paper on which the negative comments have been written and tossing it out has therapeutic benefits as well.

11. Create an action plan for handling the person or situation in an ideal manner. Maintaining mindfulness focus may help put you into flow, resulting in an improved plan of action.

12. Rehydrate or fuel your body with a healthy snack. If you focus on eating or drinking, the brain cannot continue to ruminate and rerun negative thoughts.

Enhance each of these techniques by integrating them with purposeful breathing. Additionally, your results speed up when using purposeful breathing in conjunction with these moving into mindfulness techniques.

CHAPTER 9

More Mindfulness Techniques

Most of us already have tightly packed schedules. So, where is the time available to add in some mindfulness practices throughout the workday?

Fortunately, you do not necessarily need to free up vast quantities of time during the day to practice being mindfully present. This chapter will provide a few ways to add mindfulness to what you are already doing, and none of these require more than five to ten minutes to implement.

As always, it starts with breathing. Just breathing a little deeper for a few respiratory cycles at a time reduces any stress signals coursing through your body. Do this repeatedly several times a day and you will notice improvements in your attention span and stress levels. If necessary, use a smartphone app to send you random messages throughout the day to breathe deeply (purposeful breathing).

Awareness of your posture is another way to be mindful. Are you sitting up straight or slouching? Is your neck being strained? Are your leg muscles tight? Noticing the tension in your body can make you realize that you are unconsciously worried about something that you might not have realized was troubling you.

Improving your posture is wonderful, but becoming aware of a hidden concern is even better.

Your Non-Stop Brain

You are with yourself all day long, from the time you wake up until the moment you drift off to sleep. Throughout your awake period, your mind is continuously sending you thoughts, wave after wave of seemingly random thoughts. Wouldn't it be wonderful to occasionally put these waves of thoughts on pause?

We have roughly 50,000 to 70,000 thoughts a day. Many of them, unfortunately, are not of the useful kind. And far too many of them create stress or anxiousness in us.

If we are not careful and conscious about our thoughts, these unhelpful contemplations and deliberations are likely to impact our decision-making processes, interpersonal relationships, and self-confidence.

How do you catch these unwanted and non-beneficial thoughts in action? How do you prevent them from overriding your emotional controls and paralyzing you from making decisions and taking appropriate actions? The formula is straightforward, though not easy to implement, as it likely deviates from your routine, autopilot thinking practices:

1. Become consciously aware of your thoughts. Stop and observe the thoughts running inside your mind. This is especially important when you are in an emotionally-charged situation, or when struggling with an important decision.

2. Recognize, identify, and label unhelpful thoughts. Ask yourself: *is this thought serving my best interests and purpose? Is this thought*

coming from a rational and helpful place, or is it being driven by emotions or ego?

By labeling an unhelpful thought as negative, unconstructive, useless, or obstructive, you start to lessen its power on your decision-making process and your emotional response triggers. Let such thoughts go.

3. Select your best thoughts. The ones that are helpful, conclusive, rational, constructive, useful, and enabling. This does not mean only choosing rose-colored, idealistic, and positive thoughts. This is not a "don't worry, be happy" approach. But since you can choose which thoughts to focus on, it makes sense to use the more helpful, supportive, and empowering ones.

4. Bring forth positive self-talk. It never hurts to give yourself a little self-motivation or positive reminders now and then. It may seem unnatural at first to be telling yourself *I am capable* or *I know how to make smart and realistic decisions*. But doing so becomes natural and automatic over time.

Our brains are powerful and potent. It is our choice whether we use this power to make our professional and personal lives better or worse. But we can only consciously make this choice after we routinely become aware of our thoughts and then select which thoughts are going to dominate our thinking, emotional reactions, and decision-making processes.

The brain repeats behaviors that are rewarding. When given a choice between two behaviors — one that is rewarding and one that is not — the brain will instinctively select the rewarding one.

If we pay attention to the dissatisfaction we feel when we are distracted, and compare this feeling to the positive feelings experienced when we are present, we can train our brains to see the relative rewards of each state. The more we practice this, the more we can train our brains to fend off distractions for the more rewarding experience and feeling of being mindfully present.

Other Mindfulness Techniques

Eating is another of those daily tasks we often handle on autopilot. And like most everything else done in a habitual, unthinking mode, eating provides an opportunity to pause, become centered and present, and switch into mindfulness.

A lot is written these days about mindful eating practices. I do not think you need to go all Zen with your lunch each day. On the other hand, taking a few minutes to savor several bites without thinking about email and without glancing through social media or news sites is an excellent mindful practice, especially if you are eating at your desk.

Speaking of lunch, why not have a relaxing lunch break a couple of times a week? Eat outside if possible and comfortable. Incorporate a short 15-minute stroll into the lunch period. Find a quiet place to sit with your thoughts (without judgment) for 10-15 minutes. Whatever you do, be sure to do it without any electronic devices — no checking email, text messages, social media, or calendars. The point is to find a few minutes a couple of times a week for some peace and quiet, something that very few of us have often enough.

In addition to breathing purposefully, you can enter mindfulness by walking with purpose. For most, the point of walking, particularly at work, is simply to get from one place to another. Change that by turning walks, even short ones, into opportunities to check-in with yourself: any tension spots in the body? Is your breathing shallow or deep? Are you currently mind full or mindful? What's the single most important thought you should be having at this moment? What has happened in the past 24 hours for which you are grateful?

Focusing on core listening skills is another way to become more mindful. Listening mindfully means giving full attention to not only what is said, but also to the emotions behind what is said. Listening in a mindful mode helps detect how strongly a person believes what she or he is saying.

Being fully present in the conversation also enables you to pick up on what is not being said, as well as on any hidden agendas in the room. Additionally, listening mindfully helps prevent you from interrupting colleagues or direct reports, resulting in higher levels of satisfaction, happiness, and employee engagement.

Those who practice mindfulness while listening are also more likely to be receptive to original ideas and new information. This openness creates a culture of collaboration and cooperation and results in increased innovation and better decision making.

Some people use personal mantras or favorite sayings to push themselves into mindfulness moments throughout the day. These can be pithy sayings like "happiness begins with me," or motivational messages such as "I am competent, capable, and ready to handle today's challenges."

Others might be simple reminders of deep-seated beliefs. For instance, one of my smartphone apps sends me the message *I am moving forward* at random intervals throughout the day. It also sends me several times a day the message *Am I Mind Full or Mindful?* Seeing these messages reminds me to pause, take a few deep, purposeful breaths, and refocus my thoughts on the tasks that are indeed propelling me forward.

Mindfulness at Work

Practicing mindfulness at work can help you navigate interpersonal relationships and expectations to achieve optimal results or progress. It also helps you understand and accept that you may not always get the results desired or anticipated. The key is that mindfulness is a foundation for effective work and optimal performance, and for your interactions with others.

The workplace is rife with harsh and tense conversations that bring forth an array of emotions. Mindfulness can help to alleviate the temptation to unleash an emotional outburst through a technique called anchoring. Anything you can do to focus on your physical presence and your senses is a form of anchoring. Planting your feet firmly into the floor and observing how that feels is one example. As is pushing your lower back firmly into the lumbar support area of a chair. Some people simply cross their fingers, clasp their hands, or clench their fists (beneath a table or desk, out of sight of others) as a physical reminder to regulate emotional reactions.

Another method for handling tough conversations is to stand up and walk around the room a bit. This activates the thinking part of the brain (prefrontal cortex).

Workplace stress and pressures cause tension to build up in our muscles. Here is a method for releasing and relaxing muscle tension. The key to this technique is to deliberately tense your muscles so that they will completely relax after this exercise.

> Find a comfortable place to sit, preferably in a quiet location. Remove your shoes if possible.
>
> Start with the muscles in your forehead and scalp. Take a deep breath and then tense all the muscles

in this area to a count of four. Relax the muscles as you exhale.

Continue this tensing and releasing process, coupled with deep breathing, down to other areas in your body that feel tense or sore. Mentally travel throughout your whole body, from the top of your head to the tips of your toes. Pay particular attention to the classic stress accumulation points such as neck, shoulders, jaw, middle of the back, lower back, and feet.

To be purposeful and creative, you need to create space for yourself.

Here are some other ways to incorporate mindfulness practices in the workplace. It is unlikely that you will want to use all of these, so simply pick a few that suit your lifestyle and working conditions. Most of these techniques take five minutes or less, and some work nicely in conjunction with activities that you are already doing.

1. Take two bites of food or two sips of a hot beverage. Focus on the sensory experiences of taste, smell, texture, temperature, and even the appearance of the food.

2. Take two deep breaths using the 4-7-8 purposeful breathing method (page 131). What sensations stir in your body? How do these breaths make your shoulders, nostrils, and abdomen feel?

3. Remove your shoes and place feet firmly on the floor. Stretch your toes upward as far as you can while inhaling deeply. Feel the stretch of your feet and calf muscles. Relax the toes as

you exhale. Now raise your heels as high as you can while taking another deep breath. Note the stretch in your feet and leg muscles. Relax heels as you exhale.

4. Spend a minute observing nature through a window. Which trees are fluttering in the wind? Any animals about? What images do the shadows make? Which spot looks the most peaceful?

5. Go outside and feel the warmth of the sun and the flow of the air on your skin. How does your body react to this warmth? Can you bring the warmth into your body with a deep breath? Does the feel of the sun on exposed skin make you feel energized?

6. Sit comfortably, close your eyes, and mentally scan your body from toes to head. Where is there discomfort? Pain? Relaxation? Take two deep purposeful breaths while conducting this body scan.

7. Get into a comfortable sitting position, spine straight, and, if possible, shoes off. Spend ten seconds noticing any tension, pain, or pressure points in your body. Then bring both arms straight above your head while inhaling deeply. Be sure to inflate the abdomen first, then your lungs. Hold your breath for three to five seconds while physically tensing every part of your body, from head to toes. Release the tension as you exhale and lower the arms to your side. As you exhale, focus your awareness

on the tension releasing from your body. Repeat this process three to four more times with an unrushed, steady pace.

8. Add two or three things to your gratitude list. What are you grateful for in your life? What good things have happened in the past 12-24 hours? These can be simple things, such as an unusually easy commute to work this morning, or the way sunlight feels warm on a chilly day.

9. Spend a minute reading your gratitude list from the past three to four days. Alternatively, think about something you look forward to doing later in the day or week. Studies have shown that the brain physically changes when gratitude becomes a habit. And a quick reminder of the things you are thankful for will put you in a better frame of mind as you prepare to tackle that next task or go into the next meeting.

10. Stop. Observe. Absorb. Simply stop whatever you are doing or thinking for 60 seconds and pay full attention to what is happening around you. Who appears to be on the edge of anger or frustration? Who is fully focused and concentrated on their work? What is the emotional mood of the room?

11. Stop. Observe. Reflect. Simply stop whatever you are doing or thinking for 60 seconds and pay full attention to your emotions, physicality, and thought patterns. Are you feeling tired? Stressed? Are you on the precipice of anger or frustration? What has occupied your mind the

most for the past hour or two that you have not handled or delegated? What is keeping you from being fully present in the moment? Write these things down and then set them aside (or tackle them immediately).

12. For one minute, concentrate only on slowly opening and closing your fists, while breathing deeply. Notice how tension in your hands and arms dissipates each time a fist opens.

13. Spend one minute mentally recapping the key points from a meeting or conversation that just concluded. What actions were agreed? What points are still unclear? How do you feel about the conversation or meeting? What improvements would you suggest for the next time this interaction takes place?

14. Send someone mental compassion. Think of someone you want to express compassion for, and then mentally send them some vibes of compassion. Doing so makes you less caught up in your own worries and concerns. Plus it feels good, especially if you follow up later in person with some physical or verbal compassion.

15. To overcome the hazards of sitting too long, give your body a little twist now and then. Start by placing your feet on the floor, approximately in line with the outer points of your shoulders. As you breathe out, slowly and gently rotate your rib cage to one side. It usually helps to bring the hand on the side you

are rotating across your body to its opposite shoulder. Your elbow should point down and line up approximately level with your navel. Hold this position for three to five seconds. As you inhale, bring yourself back to the center and elongate your spine by sitting tall. With the next breath out, slowly and gently twist to the other side, hold for three to five seconds, and then return to center as you inhale. You can easily complete three or four cycles of this exercise within a minute.

This twisting exercise is a healthy internal compression, which gently stretches the muscles near your rib cage while also squeezing your kidneys, spleen, liver, and other organs. As you unwind from these twists, fresh new oxygen, blood, and nutrients are pumping into these organs and the surrounding tissues. It also stretches back muscles that have become stagnant and sore from too much sitting.

16. Stop staring at the computer screen. Look away at anything else (except a handheld electronic device or mobile phone) for 40 seconds or longer. This helps to reboot the brain and also refreshes the eyes.

17. Slip on your earbuds and listen to a quick guided meditation from a smartphone app. There are hundreds to choose from and most are free, though some do have monthly membership fees attached. You will find a few of my favorites listed in the Appendix.

18. Watch relaxation sites on the Internet, like rainymood.com and simplynoise.com play soothing sounds that encourage you to relax and unwind.

19. Eat a raisin with full concentration and focus — what does the raisin look like? How does it feel in your hand? What does it smell like? What does it taste like? How does it feel on the tongue and against your gums? How long does it take for you to chew it slowly before swallowing? This may seem silly, but I guarantee you it will take your mind off any other thoughts and prepare you to be mindfully present and re-engage.

20. Sniff some essential oils. Studies show that certain scents can have a significant impact on your cortisol levels, your mood, and your productivity. Pleasant scents to use for relaxation or unwinding are lavender, peppermint, and bergamot.

Here are some other ways to gain mindfulness, but these take a little more effort and time than the techniques above:

1. Find some nature. The Japanese practice of *Shinrin-yoku* is known in English as "forest bathing." Research shows that spending some time in nature significantly reduces cortisol and blood pressure while boosting parasympathetic brain activity, the part of the nervous system responsible for rest and equilibrium.

2. Go for a walk for at least 15 minutes, and preferably for 20-30 minutes. This helps to

reduce the effects of depression and also allows you to focus on other things besides the ones troubling and stressing you.

3. Start each morning by taking five to ten minutes to establish your intentions for the day. Setting your intentions will help to clear your mind and create a sharp focus on how to proceed mindfully throughout the day. Methods for setting your intentions include reading, meditation, journaling, or light stretching and body movement.

4. Color a picture. Adult coloring books are a peaceful way to spend agonizing periods (such as sitting on a plane or in a doctor's waiting room), and it is amazing how focused and "locked-in" this enjoyable activity can be.

5. Go grocery shopping. Forcing your brain to work through a shopping list turns off mental chatter and negative thoughts.

6. Exercise for 15-30 minutes. Walking, jogging, swimming, weight lifting, stretching, rowing machine, or treadmill. It does not matter, as long as it forces you to concentrate on the activity with a singular focus.

7. Do yoga for 15-30 minutes. Most yoga practices incorporate elements of both breathing and mindful concentration.

8. Do a crossword or Sudoku puzzle, both of which take enormous concentration and focus.

9. Count backward from 500 using different intervals, such as by four, seven, eight, or nine.

At first, this may seem tedious, but the harder it becomes, the more you will need to concentrate.

10. Listen to music and fully concentrate on the lyrics. What are the meanings behind the words and phrases used?

11. Close your eyes and visualize something pleasant, peaceful, or calm. Within seconds you will undoubtedly feel a slight smile start to unfold. That is a sign that stress and anxiety are reducing.

12. Prepare a meal from scratch. Even after a stressful day at work — perhaps even most after a stressful day — washing, chopping, mixing, and tasting ingredients helps to tune out stress. It also helps to be a little creative, so change the recipe a bit or try matching different food combinations you have not tried before.

13. Clean your house, focusing on one chore at a time — mirrors, floors, vacuuming, dusting, etc. This is not the most fun activity, but the rewards are reduced stress and a cleaner house to enjoy.

14. Brush your teeth while paying attention to the entire brushing process.

15. Listen to a guided meditation. There are hundreds of apps and websites containing guided meditations of various lengths (see the list in the Appendix).

16. Journal your thoughts, including why you are feeling a certain way and what your thoughts are about these feelings.

17. Maintain a gratitude journal by noting five to seven things every day for which you are thankful and grateful. Research has shown that this simple activity is an immediate mood booster. It also helps to be very specific when journaling your gratitude thoughts. Rather than write, "I am grateful for the love of my partner," be specific, such as "I am grateful for the way my partner expressed their love for me by taking the time to listen to what I had to get off my chest today."

18. Practice mindful observation by selecting any object and giving it your full attention. How would you describe the texture and the color of the object? How well does it fit in the room, or does it feel out of place? Where do you think it was made? Why?

19. Read a book for at least half an hour, with your phone and all other electronic devices set to airplane mode. Just concentrate on the story and plot if it is a fiction book, or on the topic and subject matter if it is a nonfiction book.

In the next chapter, we will share with you a range of mindfulness meditation techniques that you can implement both in the office and at home.

CHAPTER 10

Mindfulness Meditation Techniques

Getting into a daily routine of mindfulness meditation is extremely easy, particularly with the number of meditation tools, apps, and books on the subject.

Frankly, all it really takes is a little knowledge on the subject plus commitment and resolve on your part to set aside 10-15 minutes a day. Once you get started, you are likely to find the experience so enjoyable that you will quickly increase your daily practice to around a half hour.

One caveat though: mindfulness meditation is not something you simply add to your daily to-do list and then cross it off once you complete your session. Do not treat meditation as another daily task or chore. You must meditate with heartfelt desire so that you can take its benefits with you throughout the day.

Mindfulness meditation is basically a systematic way to slow down your thoughts enough so that you can effectively watch them. Meditation is not about trying to stop thinking. It is about observing your thoughts from a nonjudgmental perspective.

Learning how to meditate is a continuous cycle of observing your thoughts, getting distracted by a thought, regaining focus, and returning to observing them. Points of focus, such as a phrase or object, are used to slow down the entry of random thoughts and give the meditator something to bring their attention back to when they catch their minds wandering.

Meditation

Perhaps the best way to get control over our thoughts is through regular mindfulness meditation practice. Think of mindfulness meditation as an excellent way of developing and strengthening your mental fitness — an exercise regimen for your brain.

For a mindfulness meditation session, there are a couple of posture practices I recommend. First, get comfortable either sitting up straight or in a reclined position. A good rule to remember is "the health of the spine determines the health of the body." As I find it uncomfortable and impossible to sit on futons and floor pillows, I either sit in a lounge chair, on the couch, or lie down on the bed. You will also frequently find me meditating while sitting in an airplane, with a noise-canceling headset covering both ears.

As you begin, relax every part of your body, starting with the toes and calf muscles. Work your way up to your jaw and the tiny muscles around your eyes. Be sure to relax your shoulders and tip your chin slightly forward toward your chest to lengthen and stretch your neck muscles. All this bodywork takes place while inhaling deeply, pausing for a couple of seconds, and then exhaling completely.

There are three main formats for mindfulness meditation:

> Open monitoring — place your mental focus on observing the content of your thoughts in a nonjudgmental and non-reactive way to become reflectively and pensively aware of cognitive and emotional patterns.
>
> Focused attention — placing sustained focus and attention on a particular object, thought, mantra, or image. When the mind wanders, purposefully bring focus and attention back to the object, thought, mantra, or image.
>
> Self-transcending — uses a mantra, often Sanskrit sounds, which the meditator can attend to without effort or concentration. The goal is for the mantra to become secondary and ultimately disappear as self-awareness increases.

When practicing mindful meditation regularly (daily is best) and consistently, we create what authors Daniel Goleman and Richard Davidson call "altered traits." They describe these mental states in their book *Altered Traits: Science Reveals How Meditation Changes Your Mind, Body, and Brain* as:

> "lasting changes or transformation of being, and they come classically through having an altered state through meditation, which then has a consequence for how you are day-to-day — and that's different than how you were before you tried the meditation."

Engaging in regular meditation trains your mind to focus awareness on the present and brings a state of calmness and peacefulness into your life. This state is more than just a good feeling; it is also good for your health as well. Meditating benefits your body in many ways, including:

- Improving mental health through stress reduction
- Boosting mood
- Reducing risks for depression
- Reducing harmful inflammation throughout the body
- Greater control of food cravings, particularly for unhealthy foods and snacks
- Preventing or slowing premature aging
- Staving off colds
- Reducing sensitivity to pain

Likewise, mindfulness meditation has direct benefits for your brain as well:

- Helping maintain the health of the brain
- Slowing natural brain aging
- Decreasing mind wandering
- Increasing the ability to concentrate and focus
- Reducing symptoms of depression and anxiety
- Enhancing brain volume and cortical thickness
- Aiding in addiction recovery

As in the previous chapter on Mindfulness Techniques, the key to successful mindful meditation is to get comfortable in a quiet place where you are unlikely to be disturbed. Set the timer on your smartphone to the desired length for your meditation session. I started at only eight minutes, then gradually increased this period in two-minute increments every couple of days.

Once you are ready, begin to focus your attention on purposeful breathing, trying not to think of anything but the air going into and out of your body. When you first start to meditate, your monkey brain is likely to be full of scattered, often unconnected thoughts. Just let these thoughts enter your mind and then send them away with each breath exhalation.

Meditation Techniques

Most meditation guides will instruct beginners to focus only on their breathing patterns. This is good advice, but often easier to understand than to actually follow. I suggest you start out this way, and then within a couple of minutes, switch your focus to any one thing that works for you: a single thought, a color, surrounding sounds, or even a mantra or word phrase that has meaning to you. The key objective is to slow down the incoming scattered thoughts until they are all but completely halted.

One suitable meditation technique for beginners is called the body scan meditation. With eyes closed and purposeful breathing in place, develop a mental scan of how your body feels. Let each part of your body "talk" to your brain by concentrating on these internal body signals.

Start with your feet and toes. Pay full attention to these (and only these) for a few moments. Lightly stretch your feet and toes and notice the sensations this causes. Move upward to your ankles and calf muscles. Again, focus for a few moments then stretch lightly. Continue progressing through your knees, upper legs, hips, pelvic region, abdomen, chest, shoulders, and neck. Then move outward along your arms down to your hands and fingers. Finish with your facial muscles and lips.

Another meditation technique I practice I call the Sunlight Bath Meditation. This is best performed just after sunrise when the warmth of the sun's rays are strong, but not overwhelming or at intense levels of ultraviolet concern.

In this meditation, I sit comfortably in a spot where the sun will directly wash my face for five to seven minutes. With eyes closed, I focus on the warmth of the sun and how its yellow rays bathe my eyelids. Taking several long and deep breaths, I settle in and imagine my body surrounded by this yellow light — a light full of solar energy and power.

I then begin to purposefully breathe in this energy with deep breaths, mentally following the energy into my diaphragm and lungs. With each subsequent deep inhalation, I breathe this energy into other parts of my body (feet, legs, abdomen, arms, etc.). Finally, I take three to four consecutive deep breaths and "breathe" this solar energy into my brain — holding each breath for a count of 12 or longer. This usually results in a "white-out" visual sensation within my mind as the solar energy swirls around my brain.

I incorporate the Sunlight Bath Meditation into my longer meditative sessions, especially during autumn and spring, when the warm sunlight feels so good in the morning coolness. I find it to be especially invigorating and energizing.

Another mindful meditation technique is a free-form session, where you simply allow thoughts to appear in your mind at free will. Rather than concentrating on any particular thought or sound, in this meditation you patiently permit any and all thoughts and images to pop up uncontrolled.

Focus on becoming aware of the moment when each thought or image appears. As these surface, watch them for a few moments without trying to force them away. Notice how these thoughts rise and fall like waves across your brain. See which thoughts last longest, and which thoughts trigger other thoughts.

The key here is to observe your thoughts and pictures patiently, without judgment or emotion. Let them enter and go, rise and fall, uninterrupted, and without a response from you. With practice, you will notice how thoughts melt away when you stop reacting, judging, or criticizing them. At first, you may worry about "losing" some thoughts that you want to keep. Don't worry; they are not lost or gone forever. They have just moved on since they did not get a rise or response from you.

Another type of popular method for meditating is called a guided meditation. In a guided meditation, an instructor or practitioner talks you through a meditative session. These can be done in person, online, or through a range of smartphone and tablet apps.

Using a calming voice, the guided meditation leader helps you engage in visualization techniques and mental imagery to help you maintain focus during the session. Soft music or soothing sounds often play in the background behind their comforting voice.

Guided meditations are often a great way to get started with meditating, especially since there are hundreds of free guided meditation sessions available on the Internet. One source I particularly like is the website of the UCLA Mindful Awareness Research Center. It has a range of guided meditation sessions in both English and Spanish, each of which runs between three and 19 minutes.

Another good source for free guided meditations is the website of the Chopra Center. These are a bit longer (most are 13 to 28 minutes) and are thus more suited for someone with a bit of meditation experience rather than for those just starting on a mindfulness meditation journey.

Slowing Your Thoughts

For most of us, the most challenging aspect of mindfulness meditation is learning how to slow down or control our thoughts.

Actually, trying to control one's thoughts during meditation is a bit of a misnomer. Slowing them down? Definitely possible. Completely controlling them? A bit on the impossible side, though some regulation is attainable.

The truth is, our thoughts never really stop. However, through mindfulness meditation, we can reduce the intensity, speed, and loudness of our thoughts. And, most important, we can begin to exercise greater control over our actions and decisions by regulating how we respond to our thoughts.

If you try to block your thoughts from creeping into your meditation session, you will undoubtedly end up chastising yourself in frustration. When the mind wanders, allow it to do so momentarily. But rather than focus or concentrate on these thoughts — and then react to them, as is our typical behavior -- return focus to your breathing or your single predetermined meditative thought (color, word, sounds, etc.). Allow any intruding thoughts or emotions to pass through your mind.

Rather than trying to control which thoughts surface, focus on slowing down the speed at which your thoughts enter your consciousness during meditation. Remember, the brain can concentrate fully on only one thought at a time, so the more you concentrate on your predetermined meditative thought, the less frequent will be the intruding thoughts generated by your wandering mind. The secret to controlling your thoughts during meditation is in not controlling them. Let them enter slowly. Observe them. Notice them. Then let them slip away or segue into the next thought.

The better you get at not fighting against your thoughts, the sooner you will notice them slipping away. By anchoring yourself in the present moment through focusing on your predetermined meditative thought, combined with purposeful breathing and mental stillness, you will start to become rooted in your true essence. And you will understand your thoughts to be nothing more than mere thoughts, not as truths or facts. The best way to control your thoughts is to observe them without judgment or emotion.

As this happens, you will gain a sense of prevailing peace and tranquility. While this will likely be only for short moments at first, through additional practice and lengthier meditative sessions, these feelings of peace and tranquility will last longer and longer.

By becoming an active observer of your thoughts, you achieve true mental power. You realize you are bigger — and more integrated, complicated, and complex — than your thoughts and emotions. You also realize that your thoughts and emotions need not have power over you. Instead, you can exercise purposeful power over your thoughts and emotions. You can be in control.

Your thoughts, and the speed at which they surface, do not define or determine how "good" you at practicing mindful meditation. This is not a competitive activity, nor is it a zero-sum game. Some days your meditation sessions will fly by with ease. On other days you will struggle to stay mentally focused and still. Accept both experiences non-judgmentally.

Over time, your relationship with your thoughts will change, especially the more you engage in mindfulness meditation. Non-judgment and non-attachment to your thoughts increases with the cumulative time spent meditating. And, with time and practice, your intruding thoughts will rise at a slower pace. Eventually, you may reach a point when you become capable of stopping your thoughts entirely for extended periods. I am sure you can sense what it would be like to experience the peace and tranquility of such an occurrence.

One other caveat: do not think you can use meditation to withdraw from reality or to escape from the bustle and whirl of daily life. While meditation will give you a respite from the stresses caused by reality and our non-stop world, you cannot turn meditation into a channel of abandonment from reality. Unless, of course, you decide to become a meditative monk and move into a monastery.

Also, be forewarned that mindfulness meditation can become a bit addictive if practiced wrongly. As Jon Kabat-Zinn has noted, "You might be tempted to avoid the messiness of daily living for the tranquility of stillness and peacefulness. This, of course, would be an attachment to stillness, and like any strong attachment, it leads to delusion. It arrests development and short-circuits the cultivation of wisdom."

Go forth and use mindfulness meditation as both a scientifically proven stress releaser and as a conduit for the cultivation of wisdom.

Your result will be: Better Decisions. Better Thinking. And Better Outcomes.

CHAPTER 11

It's Up To You

No longer solely associated with an alternative lifestyle culture, mindfulness and meditation are daily practices used by millions of people around the globe, including corporate executives, celebrities, entrepreneurs, college students, teachers, professional athletes, and just about every other job category imaginable.

Notably, the top download in 2017 in the Apple App Store was the meditation app Calm. Amazon lists over 1000 books on mindfulness. Corporations are adding mindfulness to their employee wellness programs. Children are taught mindfulness in school as a way of controlling anger. Mindfulness is going mainstream, partly because of science research results and partly due to people needing and wanting a non-pharmaceutical method of stress relief and emotional control.

So, how about you? How will you incorporate mindfulness into your life, now that you have read this book?

Will you use mindfulness to control emotional hijackings? To help you make better decisions? To improve your overall health and wellbeing? The choice is up to you.

In this book, I focused on how stress and anxiety impact your decision-making processes, and thus your decisions and outcomes. But hopefully I have also given you enough information for you to sense that mindfulness not only helps with your decision making, but also in so many other ways.

Better decision making and better thinking — and thus better outcomes — can be yours by focusing on two things:

1) Reducing stress, particularly elevated and extended periods of stress, and

2) Improving the health and functioning of your brain through better eating practices, increased exercise, and mindfulness practices.

The key is to start making better decisions, such as:

Learning to respond, rather than reacting, to situations, events, and people.

Pausing to prevent emotional hijacking.

Implementing stress reduction and stress management techniques on an on-going basis.

Taking proactive steps to go from *mind full* to *mindful* throughout every day.

Increasing your daily physical activity now and continuing this throughout your retirement years.

Only you can make better decisions to reduce your stress, prevent emotional hijacking, and improve the long-term health of your brain. No one else can do this for you.

Spread the Message

In addition to taking care of yourself, you owe it to your family, friends, colleagues, and neighbors to be a conduit for the dissemination of the information and steps in this book.

At work, be a living example of a person or leader who can transition from a *mind full* state to a *mindful* one. Use the mindfulness at work practices in chapter 9 to take control of your emotions and increase your cognitive capabilities. Wow your colleagues with better thinking that results in better outcomes. And if you need help, I provide personalized 1:1 coaching on how to go from *mind full* to *mindful* decision making and leadership.

Additionally, bring in our team of expert facilitators and coaches into your organization with our workshops and customized programs. Our workshop *Better Decision Making: Shifting from Mind Full to Mindful Leadership* is built around the fundamental principles and techniques found in this book. It can be delivered both virtually and in the classroom.

Together we can make your organization less stressful, more engaging and productive, and even a happier place to work.

I am committed to providing on-going support, materials, and tools for those who genuinely want to apply the information and techniques in this book within their organizations and communities.

How you go about doing this is up to you. And I wish you great success in doing so.

APPENDIX

Recommended Resources

Meditation Apps
Buddhify

Insight Timer

Meditation Studio

Omvana

Simple Habit

Stop, Breathe & Think

Timeless

Welzen

ZenFriend

Mindfulness Apps
Breathe

Breathe2Relax

Calm

Headspace

I Am

Mindfulness Daily

3 Minute Mindfulness

Websites

BrainChangePro.com

HeartMath.org

MindBodyGreen.com

Mindful.org

PositivePsychologyProgram.com

About the Author

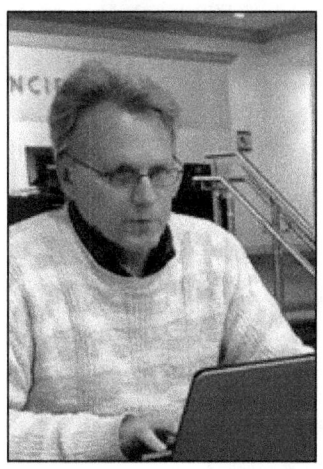

Steven Howard is an award-winning author of 21 leadership, marketing, and management books and the editor of nine professional and personal development books in the *Project You* series.

Today he creates and delivers customized leadership training programs that focus on leadership mindset, leading people, leading people development, and leading for results. He is a Certified VILT (Virtual Instructor Led Training) Facilitator, with over five years of experience running virtual leadership development programs and workshops.

In addition, Steven is an Executive Consultant with Mindful Life Training in Australia, which delivers evidence-based classroom and online training programs in decision making, mindful leadership, health and wellbeing, and mindfulness.

He specializes in creating and delivering leadership development programs for frontline leaders, mid-level leaders, supervisors, and high-potential leaders. In the past 25 years he has trained over 10,000 leaders in Asia, Australia, Africa, Europe, and North America.

Steven has delivered leadership development programs in the U.S., Asia, Australia, New Zealand, Fiji, Canada, Africa, Arabian Gulf, Europe, and Mexico to numerous organizations.

He brings a truly international, cross-cultural perspective to his leadership development programs, having lived in the USA for over 30 years, in Singapore for 21 years, and in Australia for 12 years. He currently resides in Southern California.

His other books are:

> Better Decisions. Better Thinking. Better Outcomes. How to go from Mind Full to Mindful Leadership
>
> Great Leadership Words of Wisdom
>
> 8 Keys to Becoming a Great Leader: With leadership lessons and tips from Gibbs, Yoda & Capt'n Jack Sparrow
>
> Leadership Lessons from the Volkswagen Saga
>
> Asian Words of Success
>
> Indispensable Asian Words of Knowledge
>
> Asian Words of Inspiration

Asian Words of Meaning

The Book of Asian Proverbs

Marketing Words of Wisdom

The Best of the Monday Morning Marketing Memo

Powerful Marketing Memos

Corporate Image Management: A Marketing Discipline

Powerful Marketing Minutes: 50 Ways to Develop Market Leadership

MORE Powerful Marketing Minutes: 50 New Ways to Develop Market Leadership

Asian Words of Wisdom

Asian Words of Knowledge

Essential Asian Words of Wisdom

Pillars of Growth: Strategies for Leading Sustainable Growth (co-author with three others)

Motivation Plus Marketing Equals Money (co-author with four others)

Contact Details
Email: steven@CalienteLeadership.com

Twitter: @stevenbhoward | @GreatLeadershp

LinkedIn: www.linkedin.com/in/stevenbhoward
Facebook: www.facebook.com/CalienteLeadership
Website: www.CalienteLeadership.com
Blog: CalienteLeadership.com/TheArtofGreatLeadershipBlog